C000272058

The Homœopathic
Treatment of Eczema

Robin Logan
FSHom

BEACONSFIELD PUBLISHERS LTD
Beaconsfield, Bucks, UK

First published 1998

British Library Cataloguing in Publication Data
Logan, Robin
  The homoeopathic treatment of eczema. – (Beaconsfield
homoeopathic library; no. 19)
  1. Eczema – Homeopathic treatment
  I. Title
  616.5'21'06

ISBN 0–906584–47–7

NOTICE

The names of proprietary products discussed in this book are written with an initial capital letter, whilst the generic names of products are written in small letters. The absence of any such indication does not necessarily imply that a corresponding proprietary name does not exist.

Phototypeset by Gem Graphics, Trenance, Mawgan Porth, Cornwall in 10 on 12 point Times.
Printed and bound in Great Britain by The Bath Press, Bath.

Acknowledgements

I would like to express my thanks to Nick Churchill RSHom, Bob Fordham RSHom and Dr Gabriela Rieberer MFHom for making the time to study a late draft of the manuscript for this book. Each of them gave me their detailed advice and suggestions, which I was happy to be able to take into account when preparing the final version for publication.

I would also like to thank Elizabeth Hemmings for her support, encouragement and advice, as well as my publisher John Churchill for his masterful editorial skills. I am indebted to Roger van Zandvoort for *The Complete Repertory* and to David Warkentin and Kent Homeopathic Associates for the computer version of that repertory, which has been very helpful in the creation of this book and an invaluable tool in the development of the ideas presented. Thanks are also due to all my teachers from many schools of thought, too numerous to mention.

If this book should give the erroneous impression that my cases are almost invariably successful, that was not intended and I am deeply grateful to all the people who have entrusted their health to me, whether I have been able to help them or not – they have been my most valuable teachers.

R.L.

Contents

Contents

Contents

Introduction

Eczema is notoriously difficult to treat. I believe that the reasons are not so much inherent in the condition itself but rather in our approach to treating it. If we can identify the reasons behind our failed or perplexing cases, it should be possible to develop more effective strategies for the future. It is the results of my investigations in this regard that I would like to offer here for the reader's consideration.

My main interest in homoeopathy is in striving towards an approach that seeks to understand and treat people holistically. The word 'holistic' is frequently used in connection with natural and complementary therapies. Although it has become a fashionable concept its essential meaning can easily be lost. Holistic medicine should mean more than 'treating everything'. It does not simply infer the application of a separate therapy, or in the case of homoeopathy a different remedy, for every individual complaint. Nor is it sufficient to define holism as an approach that addresses the mind, body and spirit of the person. In its deepest sense it is more than merely a form of humane, all-encompassing medicine.

To understand homoeopathy, when practised as its founder Samuel Hahnemann originally intended, is to understand the true meaning of holism. That is, we recognise the need to heal mind, body and spirit and pay attention to all the patient's symptoms, but additionally perceive the inter-relatedness of all aspects of the person and seek to make connections between seemingly disparate signs and symptoms. Good homoeopathy takes into consideration the inner world of the patient – we attempt to make sense of their emotional make-up and its often important part in the disease process.

Sometimes the patient's observable signs and symptoms take on a figurative meaning. Here the homoeopath seeks to relate the patient's inner and outer worlds in a way that involves considerable interpretative skills. Some homoeopaths are inclined to concentrate on this 'bigger picture', the emblematic patterns in the patient's symptoms, while others have a narrower perspective and concentrate more on particulars

1

and solid facts. A well-rounded practitioner needs to be conversant with both extremes, as well as every variation in between. The art lies in being able to perceive the multidimensional whole while not losing sight of the smallest details. In that way, by maintaining an open mind and a broad perspective, and by applying our inherently holistic therapy, we can exemplify holism in its most profound expression.

A classical homoeopath may, in the light of the above, wonder how a book can be written about the treatment of one particular disease. This book has contemporary classical homoeopathy as its background. That is, homoeopathy that attempts to understand the dynamics of the disease process in a holistic way, with particular regard to the role that the mind and the emotions play in the process. The recent integration of depth psychology into homoeopathic practice has been one of the most exciting developments in homoeopathy. However, trying to work in that way can at times be counterproductive – the psychosomatic approach is not appropriate in every type of case.

Even though the majority of illness is either psychosomatic, or certainly has emotional components, some of the most difficult cases are those with few or no mental symptoms. Over-reliance on mental symptoms, and attempting to make a psychological case of every patient, can lead to confusion and disappointing results. We need to be able to sense both where the centre of gravity is in the pathology of the case, as well as which elements of the information gathered from the patient are relevant to the analysis.

One of the scenarios we often encounter when treating eczema is what Samuel Hahnemann, in Paragraph 173 of the *Organon*, called 'one-sided' cases. That is, cases with very few characteristic mental and general symptoms upon which to confidently base a prescription. These cases present us with their own type of difficulties and call for particular clinical strategies. The possible reasons why eczema so often presents in this way also need to be considered. Then, having successfully analysed the case – having 'perceived what is to be cured in the patient' – we need to know how to proceed to cure, effectively adapting to any difficulties that may arise along the way.

There are several different ways in which practitioners have difficulty with eczema. Knowledge of materia medica, the techniques employed in case-taking and the intricacies of case analysis are three large subjects and a lack of skill in any of these areas will obviously limit our success. However, there are aspects of each of these subjects which relate uniquely to the treatment of eczema and which need to be understood in order to ensure satisfactory results.

The management of the eczema case also poses particular problems for many homoeopaths. In modern homoeopathic literature much emphasis is put on 'finding the remedy'. However, a suitable opening prescription does not guarantee a successful outcome. Such areas as patient education, managing and preventing aggravation, the use of topical treatment (including the influence of orthodox pharmaceutical preparations if these are part of the presenting case), dosage and, in particular, the second and subsequent prescriptions, all need to be mastered in order for treatment to be as effective as possible.

The materia medica section of this book is written with practical application in mind. The frequent use of remedies for a specific ailment allows us to develop an understanding of the essential nature of the remedy – that is, 'the person behind the symptoms' – as well as its characteristic symptoms for that complaint. Many therapeutic materia medica are of limited practical use because they present remedies as one-dimensional lists of symptoms which fail to impart any feel for the character of the remedy and what makes it unique. Precise remedy differentiations are very important in therapeutic materia medica, especially between small and polychrest remedies. I have attempted to provide a comprehensive materia medica of the remedies most relevant to the treatment of eczema in such a way as to facilitate their differentiation from other indicated remedies.

When quoting from the *Organon*, I have referred in all cases to the Sixth Edition. The repertory used throughout the book is *The Complete Repertory*, Version 3.0, by Roger van Zandvoort.

Chapter 1

Dermatology

As homoeopaths we do not require a dermatologist's knowledge of the clinical signs and symptoms of skin disease. The information given in this chapter is presented in the knowledge that much of it is not essential to the homoeopathic approach. However, an understanding of the details of the signs and symptoms of the skin can have a part to play in individualising treatment. Also, to quote James Tyler Kent in *New Remedies and Lesser Writings*, 'If you do not know sickness you are apt to think all things strange and unique.'

THE ALLOPATHIC VERSUS THE HOMOEOPATHIC VIEW

The allopathic dermatologist's view of skin disease is that there are basically two broad classifications of skin lesion:

1) Symptoms that are physiologically related to internal disease processes, e.g. erythema nodosum in leukaemia, tuberculosis or Crohn's disease.
2) Conditions considered to be 'purely dermatological', e.g. acne, eczema or psoriasis.

The difference between these classifications is that in the first group, although the skin symptoms can be an important monitor of the activity of the underlying disease, they would be of secondary importance in the evaluation of the patient. In the second group, treatment is aimed directly at the skin lesion, which is usually seen as being a purely local affection. There are exceptions to this simplification as the idea of treating disease holistically gains acceptance in the medical profession. Some skin conditions are treated with systemic medication – for example, acne with hormones. Terms such as neurodermatitis and angioneurotic oedema exist in dermatology but are not widely popular, because the connection between the mind and the skin cannot be

4

measured and is therefore subjective. Even where the influence of the psyche in skin disease is recognised, the common approach is to treat the skin symptoms directly.

Clearly this view differs from the homoeopathic one in which almost all symptoms, however superficial, are considered to be manifestations of some sort of inner disorder. The disorder may be psychological, inherited, 'miasmatic', or multi-factorial and multi-faceted, in which case it may be described as 'constitutional'. In treating the skin we are always concerned, either simultaneously or subsequently, with treating the underlying disorder.

The concept of suppression, as homoeopaths see it, does not exist in dermatology. The homoeopathic view is that the removal of peripheral symptoms by mechanical, topical or chemical means, without addressing the underlying energetic imbalance, forces the organism's defence mechanism to re-establish a state of balance. With repeated or continual suppression, the new symptoms – or imbalance – occurs on a deeper level than originally, thus affecting more important vital organs and systems in the body. Thus exterior, peripheral symptoms, when removed without addressing the underlying cause, can lead to internal, systemic disease. In allopathic medicine, the effective suppression of skin symptoms would be seen as a satisfactory outcome of treatment rather than having possibly grave consequences. The 'Law of Cure', as it is understood by alternative health practitioners, is not recognised.

Hering's Law of Cure states that cure takes place in an orderly manner and direction. Symptoms disappear from above downward, from within outward, and in the reverse order in which they occured. It is likely that the main reason why this is not acknowledged is because of conventional medicine's reluctance to make connections where there is no physiological basis for such a connection. For example, there would be no way of showing a physical connection between the suppression of an eruption and, say, mental illness or epilepsy. A homoeopath would have no difficulty in making such a connection based on our understanding of Hering's Law of Cure: that disease needs to be cured from within outwards, that during the process of cure symptoms move from more important organs to less important organs, and that the reverse of this would indicate that a harmful suppression has occurred. We model the human organism as an energetic whole, allowing for the possibility of relationships between any type of symptoms, regardless of the physiological systems in which they may arise.

There may be other factors influencing a reluctance to make

connections. One example is conventional medicine's view of the relationship between vaccination and chronic disease. The possible consequences of suggesting such relationships are profound and wide ranging.

It is assumed that any homoeopath using this book to improve their skills in the treatment of eczema is well aware of the philosophical basis of homoeopathy as promulgated by Samuel Hahnemann. Those who wish to study what he had to say about the suppression of symptoms, and of skin disease generally, should refer to paragraphs 187 to 203 of the *Organon* and the chapter entitled 'Psora' in his *Chronic Diseases*.

As already stated, the minutiae of medical classification and terminology are not of primary significance for the homoeopath. It is one of the wonders of homoeopathy that so much can be done with so little knowledge of the anatomy and physiology of the affected organ. However, it is useful and sometimes important to know exactly what you are looking at. In Paragraph 153 of the *Organon*, Hahnemann directs us to find the 'more striking, strange, unusual, peculiar symptoms in the case'. From that point of view it is important to know what is common to any disease process. The quotation from Kent's *Lesser Writings* at the beginning of this chapter can usefully be reiterated here.

Whilst it may be most important to help patients to understand their inner processes and the significance of their condition, many of them will also be familiar with the conventional medical labels relating to it. It is therefore necessary that the relevant terms are known to the non-medical homoeopath. These are referred to in the following pages.

CLINICAL FEATURES AND REPERTORY RUBRICS

Butterworths' *Medical Dictionary* defines eczema as 'A non-contagious inflammatory disease of the skin with much itching and burning. It may be acute, subacute or chronic, and takes the form of erythema with papules, vesicles or pustules that may develop into scales and crusts. It may occur at any age and may be caused by a variety of internal and external factors.'

Dermatitis is the term used for a reaction of the skin to external injury, as in 'contact dermatitis'. It is of a localised nature with a uniform appearance and usually disappears after removal of the external stimulus. The term eczema is used more often for endogenous or constitutional dermatitis. That is, dermatitis which in conventional terms has its origin within the organism. The methods of treatment described in this book can be applied to either type of skin condition, although the most common type encountered by homoeopaths is atopic eczema. Atopy is defined as the constitutional inherited tendency of some individuals to allergic hypersensitivity states, with asthma, hayfever and eczema being the principal manifestations.

There are several types of eczema defined in dermatology and for information they are discussed briefly in this chapter.

The repertory rubrics under each heading are those most closely related to that condition. They are listed mainly for the purpose of familiarising the reader with some of the useful rubrics in the skin section of the repertory. They are, however, not all complete nor very reliable rubrics. The repertory contains many descriptions and very few disease labels. For example, I have listed the rubric 'milk-crust' as the one describing cradle-cap, although there are many descriptions in the repertory that fit the complaint and which I have not listed, e.g. 'HEAD; ERUPTIONS; crusts, scabs'. Some of the rubrics have sub-rubrics that can easily be found in the repertory – for example, the rubric 'Eruptions; discharging, moist' has fourteen sub-rubrics.

Asteatotic Eczema

This has the appearance of 'crazy paving' with fissures and fine scaling and is associated with drying out of the skin. It is prevalent in old age as a result of impaired function of the sebaceous glands and less effective skin barrier.

Rubrics
    SKIN; CHAPPING
    SKIN; CRACKS, fissures
    SKIN; DRY
    SKIN; ERUPTIONS; desquamating
    SKIN; ERUPTIONS; dry
    SKIN; ERUPTIONS; scaly

Atopic Eczema

This disorder affects between one and three per cent of the population. There is a genetically predisposed tendency in families and in fifty per cent of cases it is accompanied by allergic respiratory disease. Seventy per cent of patients are aware of other family members with eczema.

Most theories suggest that atopic disease is a defect in immunology, probably depressed T-cell function and consequent lack of suppression of some aspects of antibody production. Patients with eczema usually show high reaginic (IgE) antibody levels which suggests an underlying allergic state. About eighty per cent of atopic cases react to certain foods and house dust.

The following rubrics express this connection:

Rubrics
> CHEST; ALTERNATING with; skin symptoms
> GENERALITIES; ALLERGY
> RESPIRATION; ASTHMATIC; alternating with; eruptions
> SKIN; ERUPTIONS; ALTERNATING with; asthma
> SKIN; ERUPTIONS; ALTERNATING with; respiratory symptoms

Contact Dermatitis

This is usually the result of long-term exposure to an allergen, although sensitisation can occur immediately after initial contact with a potent substance. Once sensitised, dermatitis typically appears within 48 hours of re-exposure. The most common contact dermatitis sensitisers are:

- Cosmetics. This is relatively rare now because of the lengths to which cosmetic manufacturers have gone to eliminate allergens. Hairdressers sometimes experience dermatitis caused by shampoos, conditioners and other products that they use frequently.
- Clothing. Some dyes and metal clips and buttons.
- Foods. The handling of certain foods such as some fruits, garlic and shellfish.
- Plastics, acrylic and epoxy resins.
- Plants – for example chrysanthemum, lichens and moss.
- Metals – for example, beryllium, chrome, nickel and cobalt.
- Cement dermatitis is common in builders. Calcium hydroxide is highly irritant.
- Light (eczema solare).

Rubrics
> GENERALITIES; ALLERGY
> SKIN; ERUPTIONS; friction; clothing, of; agg.
> SKIN; ERUPTIONS; sun, from
> SKIN; ERUPTIONS; vesicular; sun, from exposure to
> SKIN; SENSITIVENESS; sun, to

Eczema Papulosum

Characterised by the formation of small red papules.

Rubric
> SKIN; ERUPTIONS; papular

Eczema Pustulosum

Characterised by the formation of pustules.

Rubric
> SKIN; ERUPTIONS; pustules (many sub-rubrics)

Eczema Rubrum

This is a stage of eczema characterised by redness, swelling and infiltration. If it is red and oozing it is called eczema madidans, although this is a somewhat outdated term.

Rubrics
> SKIN; ERUPTIONS; discharging, moist
> SKIN; ERUPTIONS; eczema; madidans
> SKIN; ERUPTIONS; eczema; rubrum
> SKIN; ERUPTIONS; eczema; suppurating
> SKIN; ERUPTIONS; swelling, with

Eczema Sclerosum

The most chronic and advanced but least inflammatory eczema characterised by thickening, infiltration and lichenification.

Rubrics
> SKIN; ERUPTIONS; crusty; thick
> SKIN; HARD
> SKIN; HARD; parchment, like; dry
> SKIN; HARD; thickening, with

Eczema Siccum

Dry, scaly eczema.

Rubrics
> SKIN; DRY
> SKIN; ERUPTIONS; crusty; dry

SKIN; ERUPTIONS; desquamating; scales, white
SKIN; ERUPTIONS; dry
SKIN; ERUPTIONS; eczema; dry
SKIN; ERUPTIONS; scaly

Eczema Varicosum

Also called hypostatic eczema or gravitational eczema, arising from impaired venous return.

Rubrics
EXTREMITIES; ERUPTION; ankle; eczema; varicosum
EXTREMITIES; ITCHING; lower limbs; varices
EXTREMITIES; VARICES; leg; itching
GENERALITIES; VEINS; varicose, distended, engorged, plethoric; itching

Infantile Eczema

Most eczema sufferers develop the disease during the first nine years of life. Itching becomes apparent during the first two to six months of life. The face is usually the first site, spreading to exposed surfaces when the child begins to crawl. Secondary infection can occur after scratching. During the second year of life the most characteristic sites are the flexures of the elbows, knees, sides of neck, wrists and ankles. There is a general tendency for gradual improvement with symptoms being mild by teenage years. The breast-fed infant has about a third of the risk of eczema compared to a bottle-fed child.

Rubrics
SKIN; DRY; babies, in
SKIN; ERUPTIONS; eczema; children, in
SKIN; ERUPTIONS; eczema; dry; children, in
SKIN; ERUPTIONS; rash; children, in

Infected Dermatitis

Some eczema is related to a 'bacterial allergy', most commonly staphylococcus. This takes the form of a well-demarcated crusty, scaly patch of eczema near an ulcer or discharging wound. Infected dermatitis can also be a bacterial infection resulting from scratching. This is covered by later classifications.

Rubrics
    SKIN; ERUPTIONS; eczema; wound, in neighbourhood of
    SKIN; ERUPTIONS; vesicular; wound, around a

Nummular Eczema

Also called discoid eczema, this is the term given to eczema that has round, symmetrical lesions. They can be scattered over the whole body but are most common on the legs and are intensely itchy. They are usually vesicular and endogenous, i.e. external factors play little part in their development.

Rubric
    SKIN; ERUPTIONS; patches

Pityriasis Alba

This is a type of eczema common in darker skins, in which dry eczema gives rise to white, round or oval patches on the skin. It is common in children and adolescents.

Rubrics
    SKIN; DISCOLORATION; white
    SKIN; ERUPTIONS; colour; whitish
    SKIN; ERUPTIONS; crusty; white
    SKIN; ERUPTIONS; desquamating; scales, white
    SKIN; ERUPTIONS; rash; white
    SKIN; ERUPTIONS; scaly; white

Seborrhoeic Dermatitis

This affects areas of sebaceous activity like the neck, axillae and groin. It also involves hairy areas including the scalp and eyebrows. Marginal blepharitis and dandruff are types of seborrhoeic dermatitis. Otitis externa is another manifestation. This is usually a dull, greasy eruption.

    'Cradle cap' – thick yellow crusts and scaling of the scalp which infants develop during the first month of life, is another example.

Rubrics
    HEAD; DANDRUFF
    HEAD; ERUPTIONS; milk crust
    HEAD; SEBORRHOEA
    EAR; ERUPTIONS; eczema

EAR; ERUPTIONS; eczema; meatus
EYE; ERUPTIONS; eyebrows, about
EYE; ERUPTIONS; lids, on; margins
EYE; INFLAMMATION; lids; margins
SKIN; ERUPTIONS; hairy parts, on
SKIN; ITCHING; hairy parts

ALLOPATHIC TREATMENT

Although it is recognised that atopic eczema is not just a local condition and that there is an immunological aspect to it, the conventional treatment of eczema is almost entirely in the form of topical therapy. This is in the form of emollients, steroid creams and antipruritics. It is now recognised that these treatments have been overprescribed with resulting systemic side effects and atrophy of the skin, but they remain the only help that orthodox medicine can offer.

Topical Steroids

The issue of topical steroids is likely to arise in the homoeopathic evaluation for two reasons.

In the first place, their use will cause suppression to a greater or lesser degree, depending on their strength, and the homoeopath will need to take this into account in the management of the case. A large number of topical steroids are available, falling into four main categories – mild, moderate, potent and very potent. Individual products are not mentioned here as their names and availability can vary from country to country. Patients are mostly familiar with the proprietary names of the preparations which have been prescribed for them, and reference to the relevant national formulary will establish the likely extent of suppression to be expected. The issue of suppression is discussed at various further points in this book.

Secondly, patients with eczema will typically be using steroid preparations when they consult a homoeopath and they will very often ask whether it is necessary to continue doing so, or whether the dosage can be reduced. Any proposed variation should first be raised with the prescribing physician, even though in most cases patients are left to manage the use of their topical treatments themselves.

Steroids work by having several effects:

Anti-inflammatory
Decrease epidermal turnover
Decrease fibrin deposition
Decrease fibroplastic activity
Decrease phagocytic activity
Decrease prostaglandin synthesis
Immunosuppressive

They are applied in creams and ointments. Creams are water-based and have a cooling effect, and are used mostly for weeping lesions. Ointments are oil-based and chosen for their emollient and occlusive properties, and are used more for dry, scaly lesions. Lotions and washes are sometimes used for scalp conditions. The side effects of steroids are:

Bruising (vascular wall fragility)
Depigmentation
Hirsutism
Systemic absorption
Thinning of skin (dermis and epidermis)

It is acknowledged that steroids are not curative and that rebound exacerbation of the condition may occur after discontinuation of treatment. Severe cases of eczema may be controlled by systemic steroids. Apart from a few extreme cases, these are usually only used to help the patient over an acute period.

Other Treatments

Moisturisation of the skin is usually recommended, as is washing with soap substitutes based on emulsifying ointments. Moisturisation can be a useful non-suppressive palliative, especially in the early stages of homoeopathic treatment. Some of the more common emollients used are: Diprobase, E45, Oilatum, Sudocrem and Unguentum Merck. Aqueous Cream is another simple, well-tolerated emollient. Some preparations, such as Aquadrate, contain urea for the control of itching. Urea in steroid preparations aids the absorption of the steroids. Anti-histamines and chlorpromazine are also sometimes prescribed for the control of pruritis. Bath oils containing coal tar such as Balneum + Tar and Polytar are often prescribed.

Bacterial secondary infection is treated with systemic antibiotics.

It is interesting to note that modalities of relevance to homoeopaths have not gone unnoticed by allopaths. *The Oxford Textbook of Medicine* states: '... a change of climate does effect great improvement in some children. It may be exposure to sunlight or to the sea or to a mountain top.'

COMPLICATIONS

Dangerous medical complications are unusual and eczema rarely constitutes an emergency. The main complications to be aware of are:

- Erythroderma in severe exfoliative dermatitis is dangerous because it may result in failure of body temperature control and fluid loss.
- Severe infections can arise in neglected cases, resulting in cellulitis or even septicaemia.
- Patients with severe atopic eczema can develop cataracts at a young age.
- Herpes simplex and vaccination can induce severe febrile illness in atopic patients. This can result in Kaposi's varicelliform eruption, which may cause fatal encephalitis.

OTHER SKIN CONDITIONS THAT MAY RESEMBLE ECZEMA

The following diverse conditions may at certain stages of their development resemble eczema, but are in fact all of different origin and character. In some of them there may be the possibility of underlying serious disease. In such cases, if there is any question of doubt about their nature, the patient should be referred without delay for the appropriate specialist advice. In everyday practice, however, the patient seeking homoeopathic treatment for any of these conditions is most likely to have been under conventional medical care for it already.

Erysipelas
A streptococcal cellulitis, it has a well demarcated red, shiny, tender eruption. It often has vesicles and bullae. It is commonly accompanied by high fever and chills. It is recurrent in some patients.

Erythema Multiforme

An inflammatory eruption with symmetric erythematous, swollen lesions. The onset is usually sudden with papules, weals and vesicles appearing mostly on the extremities and the face. Often caused by drugs. Attacks last two to four weeks and often recur annually.

Fungal Infections

Also called dermatophyte infections, these include tinea corporis (ringworm), tinea pedis (athlete's foot), tinea capitis (ringworm of the scalp), tinea cruris (jock itch or dhobi itch). They usually produce only mild inflammation but can be very persistent. Tinea versicolor is a yeast infection characterised by white or brownish slightly scaly patches.

Ichthyosis

This is chronic dryness and scaling of the skin. It is usually congenital but can also be a sign of lymphoma in children.

Lichen Planus

A recurrent, itchy, inflammatory eruption with small angular papules that may join to form rough scaly patches. Mild to severe itching may be present. The oral mucosa are affected in 50% of patients. Children are rarely affected.

Pemphigus

An uncommon, sometimes fatal disease characterised by bullae on the skin and mucous membranes. The bullae arise from skin of normal appearance and leave a raw, denuded, maybe crusty area when they burst. They also occur in the mouth. The epidermis is easily detached from the underlying skin. Treatment is usually hospitalisation and large doses of corticosteroids.

Pruritis (Itching)

Itching may be termed a 'skin disease' or it may be a symptom of systemic disease.

The most itchy skin diseases other than eczema are: scabies, urticaria, insect bites, lichen planus, miliaria (blocked sweat ducts), pediculosis (lice), herpetiform dermatitis, and dry skin in the elderly.

Itching, as a symptom of systemic disease, occurs in: lymphoma, leukaemia, uraemia, obstructive biliary disease, polycythaemia, diabetes, hyperthyroidism and internal cancers.

Many drugs, especially the barbiturates and salicylamides, can also cause generalised itching.

Pruritis can occur during the later months of pregnancy.

It is also often of a psychogenic aetiology, but one should be cautious before attributing generalised pruritis to such a cause.

Psoriasis

Dry, well circumscribed silvery scaling plaques of varying sizes. It is usually not itchy. The patches are accompanied by erythematous, scaling papules. It can be confused with seborrhoeic dermatitis and lichen planus.

Scabies

The itch caused by the mite *Sarcoptes scabiei*. It is characterised by intense itching, especially in bed. The lesions are the mite's burrows, seen as thin wavy lines with a small papule at one end. Once scratched, the lesions are difficult to identify as scabies and may resemble an eczematous eruption.

Scalded Skin Syndrome

Also called toxic epidermal necrolysis, this is a severe exfoliative skin infection caused by staphylococcus. It has the appearance of scalded skin. It begins with a crusty eruption, often around the nose or ear, quickly developing to widespread redness and desquamation. The skin peels off in large sheets. It progresses rapidly and may be fatal, so it is not likely to present as chronic eczema.

RELEVANT TERMS DEFINED

Areola: A reddish ring around a skin lesion.
Blepharitis: Inflammation of the edges of the eyelids.
Bullae: Blisters containing clear fluid.
Cellulitis: Inflammation of connective tissue.
Desquamation: Peeling or scaling off of the epidermis.
Emollient: A substance that softens the skin.
Erythema: Redness of the skin.
Erythroderma: Widespread erythema with scaling and infiltration.

Fibroplastic: Producing fibrous tissue in wound healing.
Furuncles: Boils.
Hirsutism: Male distribution of hair in women.
Ichorous: Thin and watery.
Infiltration: Filling by fluid or pus.
Lichenification: A thickening or hardening of the skin forming a lesion akin to lichen.
Morphaea: Scleroderma affecting one part of the skin.
Nummular: Disc-shaped (Latin *nummus*, money).
Papules: Small, circumscribed elevation of the skin.
Petechiae: Small spots caused by extravasation of blood.
Phagadenic: Ulcerative sloughing of the skin.
Phagocyte: Cell that ingests micro-organisms.
Prostaglandin: Fatty acids found in body tissue.
Psychogenic: Originating in the mind.
Prurigo: Itching papular eruption.
Reagin: Antibody-like substances responsible for allergic reactions.
Rhagades: Fissures, particularly of anus and angle of mouth.
Roseola: Rose-coloured rash.
Rupia: Pustular eruption seen in secondary syphilis.
Scleroderma: Systemic sclerosis affecting the organs and skin.
Sebaceous: Fatty, greasy, secretion.
Serpiginous: Creeping from one surface to another.
Siccum: Dry (Latin *siccare*, to dry).
Strophulus: Prickly heat.
Sudamina: Small vesicles formed in the sweat ducts.
Vesicle: Blister.
Wen: Sebaceous cyst of the scalp.

COLLABORATION WITH THE PATIENT'S GENERAL PRACTITIONER

Many patients who consult a homoeopath will already be under the care of their general practitioner or a dermatologist. Wherever possible it is important to communicate with the physician concerned. Firstly, it is improper for a second party to interfere with the treatment prescribed by the first party without his or her knowledge. Secondly, successful homoeopathic treatment will almost certainly lead to the modification and probable reduction of the conventional medication, and the original prescribing doctor should be made aware of this.

Even though many patients increasingly come to the homoeopath in the first instance rather than as a last resort, the need for communication remains. The most satisfactory situation is one in which the homoeopath has an open relationship with the patient's general practitioner or consultant, keeping him or her informed of the patient's progress.

However, this is an ideal which cannot always be achieved. Many conventional doctors are sceptical of homoeopathy and some are actually hostile towards it. Attempts at communication in such instances are usually fruitless. Furthermore, some patients will not want to tell their GP that they are having homoeopathic treatment, and this too needs to be respected.

Another reality in the matter is that chronic eczema patients are frequently given repeat prescriptions of conventional medicines over long periods, and are more or less left to manage the condition and its treatment by themselves. Hydrocortisone is also now available in the UK as an over-the-counter medicine, which is an indication of the conventional view of its suitability for self-administration.

It is always worth the effort of making contact with the patient's GP, and not just for the reasons above. More and more conventional doctors are becoming interested in homoeopathy, and we have an important role to play in making them more aware of what it has to offer.

Chapter 2

Taking the Case of an Eczema Patient

This book assumes that the reader is competent in basic homoeopathic skills. Intrinsic to those skills should be the ability to take a thorough case history. Most of this chapter focuses on gathering information relevant to the treatment of eczema by the methods explained later. It is not the intention to provide instruction in the rudiments of case-taking. However, some aids to improving general case-taking technique are included.

STARTING WITH PARTICULARS

In certain eczema cases, and in particular severe ones, it is useful to begin taking the case by investigating the presenting complaint in as much detail as possible. There are two chief reasons why it is helpful for case notes to begin with a precise description of the presenting condition:

1) As will be seen in the next chapter, a detailed understanding of every aspect of the skin symptoms can play an essential part in the analysis of the case and the selection of the second prescription.
2) It serves as a specific reference point from which to gauge responses to treatment. Sometimes patients will report that they are 'not better' on returning for a follow-up consultation. Taking this statement literally can be misleading and may result in the homoeopath abandoning a remedy that is acting curatively. It frequently occurs in practice that patients use an expression like 'not better' to imply they are not cured yet. Beware of being misled into thinking that they are saying that there has been no improvement at all. When symptoms disappear it is remarkable how quickly patients can forget that they ever had them. The true healing process is gentle and often unspectacular; a gradual return to normality is frequently only fully appreciated in retrospect. It is best in follow-up consultations to refer

back to the details of the original description of the complaint, to assess whether there has been an improvement or not.

Related to this is the importance of documenting the quantity of topical treatment being used. It is clearly important to know that the patient who says they are not better is using half as much hydrocortisone as usual.

It is often the case that a patient presents with a physical problem like eczema, whereas on closer examination it becomes clear to both practitioner and patient that the physical problem is a manifestation of something more complex. In those situations the presenting complaint will lose its priority status as the treatment focuses on deeper issues. However, the physical symptoms can still be a useful barometer of remedy reaction, especially where you are dealing with nebulous and changeable emotional states that can be easily influenced by life circumstances or are particularly susceptible to suggestion and the placebo effect. Also, many eczema patients will present with good energy levels but minimal mental symptoms that can be used to assess remedy reaction.

If there has been a response, the description of the complaint will serve another very important purpose. A decision will have to be made as to how to proceed – is the same remedy appropriate or is a different one required? This is also discussed in detail in Chapter 3, where it will be shown how, often, only a detailed analysis of the symptoms of the eczema will make it possible to determine the next prescription.

Another way of beginning is to list all the health problems the patient would like help with and then go through each of them in a more detailed way. If there is more than one presenting complaint it is often useful to do an overall survey before detailing particulars – this can give you an initial sense of the centre of gravity of the case and a feel for which areas require closer examination. Such an 'overall survey' can also suggest a significant pattern or theme running through the case. Certain case analysis techniques, for example, arranging symptoms into themes or seeking the common denominator that characterises all the symptoms in the case, are most successfully approached in this way. Remember, though, to allow the patient to take the lead if they are providing the momentum for the case-taking process – patients usually have their own sense of where the 'centre of gravity' is.

There are cases where the physical symptoms are not useful in the analysis and their description will occupy no more than a line or two. Sometimes there are no modalities or characteristic symptoms amongst those of the presenting complaint and here we pay more attention to the mental and general symptoms. These are usually mild eczema cases or ones in which there has been very effective suppression. This subject is also discussed more fully in Chapter 3.

Case-taking is an organic process and is as individual as the patient. In reality there are as many ways of taking the case as there are patients. The suggestions given here are offered as guidelines rather than rules.

Some prefer to describe the process as 'receiving the case' rather than 'taking the case'. This is a good way of looking at it, as we should avoid being too directive and prescriptive in our relationship with the patient. In most cases, however, it is best to do the 'receiving' once you have ascertained why the patient is consulting you and have explored every aspect of the chief complaint.

OPEN QUESTIONS

Ask the open question, 'Is there anything that markedly makes the skin better or worse?'. Apart from the more common modalities like warmth and washing, surprising replies like 'Yes, when I am angry' can be given to these open questions . The more spontaneous the answer to an open question, the more valuable the symptom. Usually, if the question has to be considered for a long time, or the answer contains 'maybe', 'sometimes', 'possibly' or similar words, the modality is less likely to be worth considering as important. As will be seen in the case analysis chapter, modalities of the skin symptoms are one of the most useful types of information. One very marked modality can eliminate a hundred remedies from the analysis, or narrow your choice down to a small workable number.

The system of underlining or grading symptoms is invaluable. A spontaneous answer to an open question would be underlined two to four times, depending on the frequency and intensity of the symptom – in other words, how reliable the symptom is. Paper cases where no such system has been used are virtually impossible to work with. A one-dimensional list of symptoms – that is, one with no hierarchy or grading – is of very limited use.

DIRECT QUESTIONS

Whether the patient has volunteered anything or not, proceed by asking direct questions about factors that affect the skin for better or worse.

Answers to direct questions are usually of less value than those to open questions. There are, however, factors that influence the importance of these symptoms. People will sometimes omit to mention something because, for example:

- They have got so used to living with the symptom or modality that they overlook it, such as a particular allergy that has necessitated giving up the food responsible. The avoidance of that food has become an integral part of their life and the aggravation from it is therefore never experienced.
- They consider the symptom to be a common experience for eczema sufferers and therefore not worth mentioning. An example of this is someone who takes an hot bath to relieve the itching, not realising that many eczema sufferers' itching is much worse for hot bathing.

Always ascertain the intensity and reliability of the modality. Only modalities underlined two or more times should be relied on in the analysis of the case. Beware of conditioned responses – a patient may have followed guidelines issued by the GP or an eczema sufferers' support group. For example, patients are often told to avoid water and overheating so as to prevent drying of the skin. Asking such a person whether their skin is worse for exposure to water may elicit a misleading response.

MODALITIES

Work your way through all the following modalities:

The Effects of:

Air
Cold
Exertion
Foods
Heat
Lack of sleep
Occupation
Perspiration
Seasons
Sleep
Time
Touch

Undressing
Washing – hot and cold
Weather
Wool

The effect of scratching: is the itch better, worse, unchanged or does it change place on scratching?

These modalities may refer to the itch, or the eruption, or both. Be clear about that in your notes.

Emotional Modalities

There are many different mental states that can aggravate or ameliorate eczema. Some of the more common ones are:

Admonition and reproaches.
Anger, the effects of expressing it, suppressing it or being subject to the anger of others.
Anticipation
Anxiety
Consolation
Contradiction
Excitement
Mental exhaustion
Occupation
Weeping – may be better or worse for shedding tears.

Again it must be stressed that these modalities have to be marked if they are to be useful. It is always important to distinguish between a modality that effects the whole person generally and one that effects the skin symptoms. This information can be useful in understanding 'layered' cases (ones which go through a sequence of indicated or 'uppermost' remedies) and differentiating between those where the constitutional remedy or a more superficial remedy may be indicated. This is discussed further in Chapter 3.

Character of Eruption

Ask about the nature of the eruption. Is it:

Desquamating
Dry
Dry but discharging after scratching
Moist

If there is a discharge, what is its character? Is the discharge:

    Bloody
    Offensive
    Pussy (purulent)
    Sticky
    Watery

What colour is the discharge?

Does the skin crack? If so, are the fissures superficial or are they deep and bloody?
Is the eruption:
    in patches?
    vesicular – singular or grouped?
Is the eruption crusty? If so, what colour are the crusts?

Sensation

Ascertain whether there is anything distinguishing about the sensation, for example:

    Biting
    Burning
    Itching, burning after scratching
    Prickling
    Stinging

Strange sensations, for example 'like a mouse running on the skin' or 'insects crawling' are sometimes reported. These sensations can be taken literally and looked up in the repertory, or may be used in a more figurative way in the analysis. This is useful where a theme suggests itself in the analysis. So, for example, a hidebound sensation of the skin where a suppressed remedy like Staphysagria is suggested could be useful; a wandering itch in a Tuberculinum case would also be characteristic.

Location

The location of the eruption can be relevant if it definitely restricts itself to one part of the body. As can be seen in the materia medica section, and by studying the repertory, you may see cases, for example, in which the eczema is only on the eyelids or only behind the ears. Some remedies have an affinity for eruptions on certain parts of the body.

Some remedies have an affinity for eczema in the flexures of the

24

joints. This is only a useful symptom if the eczema is found nowhere but the bends of the joints, since it is a common site for eczema to appear.

Bilaterally symmetric eruptions are encountered from time to time. The eruption occurs in the same place on both sides of the body at the same time. The exactness of the symmetry can be remarkable. This symptom is under-represented in the repertory but it can be exhibited in Arnica, Lac Caninum, Syphilinum and Thyroidinum.

One of the worst repertorisations I have ever seen was of an eczema patient who brought their previous homoeopath's notes. The case had been repertorised: eruptions; face, eruptions; shoulders, eruptions; hands, eruptions; behind ears, and so on. Such repertorisation, based on non-characteristic symptoms, is a waste of time. It yields many remedies, mostly polychrests, of equal (useless) rank in the repertorisation.

CONCOMITANT SYMPTOMS

Other symptoms that intensify at the same time as the skin symptoms are very important. They are part of the same energetic disturbance as the eruption and may hold clues as to the indicated remedy. There are many types of concomitant symptoms; some of the typical ones are food desires and aversions, for example the patient who craved chocolate whenever the eruption was particularly bad – a sign that together with the rest of the important symptoms of the case helped to arrive at the prescription of Sepia.

There may be a mental symptom, for example the patient suffering from urticaria who found she had a very strong desire to be alone during flare-ups – a symptom that helped to eliminate certain remedies like Arsenicum, Phosphorus and Pulsatilla. It helped to confirm Natrum Muriaticum. During severe itching it is common for the sufferer to be mentally distressed, but it is always worth investigating the state of mind of the patient at the time that the eczema symptoms are at their worst. It is at these times that unconscious emotional disturbances can surface in subtle ways, revealing something of the nature of the 'core disturbance' that may be at the root of the skin problem. These are different from the modalities mentioned above. Distinguish between exciting causes, modalities and concomitant symptoms.

There may be a simple general symptom like an increase or decrease in body temperature during exacerbation that can help eliminate a whole group of remedies. An example of this is a case with many symptoms suggesting Mezereum as the remedy. However, the patient always felt generally warmer when the eruption was bad. This contra-indicated Mezereum and was more suggestive of the main competing remedy, Sulphur. The two rubrics to compare in this regard are:

GENERALITIES; HEAT; sensation of
GENERALITIES; HEAT; vital, lack of

(Mezereum, whilst having itching that is worse from warmth, is usually very chilly.)

ALTERNATING SYMPTOMS

In the repertory the most important rubrics relating to symptoms of this sort are:

SKIN; ERUPTIONS; General; alternating with; asthma
SKIN; ERUPTIONS; General; alternating with; internal affections
SKIN; ERUPTIONS; General; alternating with; respiratory symptoms

The main remedy for eczema alternating with internal complaints is Graphites, especially with digestive symptoms like stomach ulcers. Croton Tiglium has eczema alternating with diarrhoea. The main remedies for eczema alternating with asthma are Caladium, Croton Tiglium, Graphites, Mezereum, Psorinum, Rhus Tox. and Sulphur.

It is also worth being aware of the rubric: 'Mental symptoms alter-nating with physical symptoms'. Platina is well known for this but is not the only remedy with that characteristic. From the point of view of eczema, Alumina, Belladonna and Tuberculinum can also exhibit an alternation of physical and mental symptoms.

Take care that it is a true alternation of symptoms. Periodic asthma in a patient with eczema does not constitute an alternation of symptoms. It can only be described as such if the asthma definitely coincides with periods when the eczema is better – a situation often encountered in patients who are receiving suppressive treatment of some sort.

AETIOLOGY

Aetiology is defined by Chambers Dictionary as 'the philosophy of causation: an enquiry into the origin or causes of anything, especially diseases'.

The importance of aetiology in homoeopathic case-taking and analysis is well known to practitioners. It is also known as 'never been well since', abbreviated 'nbws' in case notes. There are some aetiologies of particular relevance to eczema. Except in special circumstances, we should avoid a reductionist approach that seeks to identify individual, specific causes and bases prescriptions on aetiology alone, since this is a non-holistic, essentially allopathic view of disease causation. Rather, the aetiology should be seen as one aspect of the totality.

Vaccination as an Aetiology

This is an important but complicated subject. It is important because homoeopaths almost universally acknowledge that vaccination is potentially harmful. Many of the old texts mention it as a cause of eczema. The *Complete Repertory* lists the following remedies in the rubric 'Eruptions after vaccination': Crotalus Horridus, Malandrinum, Mezereum, Sarsaparilla, Skookum Chuck, Sulphur and Variolinum. These, and other vaccinosis remedies, are discussed in Chapter 6.

Vaccination is a difficult subject because it may often only be suspected as an aetiology. It is common for infants to develop eczema during the first six months of life, and it is unreasonable always to assume that has been caused or catalysed by vaccination. I remember once lecturing the mother of an eight-month-old infant with severe eczema on the evils of vaccination only to be told that the child had not been vaccinated! It is further complicated by the fact that there is no way of knowing which one of the immunisations is responsible. If other indications suggest a remedy like Mezereum, Sarsaparilla or Sulphur, then the suspected vaccinosis strengthens the case for that remedy.

If, however, the indications are not clear and vaccinosis is suspected, you may find yourself in the somewhat difficult position of having to prescribe several tautopathic (made from a vaccine) remedies 'blind' in the hope that one or more of them will have a curative effect. My experience of prescribing vaccinations in potency has not been very rewarding. However, this contradicts the experience of other practitioners, and is worthy of further research. I recommend using vaccine remedies on their own, and not in conjunction with other remedies, as it is otherwise impossible to assess their efficacy.

Emotional Aetiology

It is not unreasonable to believe that the majority of diseases have an emotional aetiology and I encourage thorough investigation along these lines. In the case of infants, the mother's emotional state during pregnancy is very important. It has been verified many times over by homoeopaths that a child can inherit susceptibilities other than the commonly recognised genetically inherited diseases from its parents. Actual remedy states can be passed on to the infant, especially from the mother. Where this has happened, the inherited remedy picture is usually most apparent very early on in the child's life, before its own more individual patterns take shape.

One common scenario is a Sepia state during pregnancy which 'grafts' Sepia symptoms onto the unborn foetus, resulting in Sepia eczema. It is by this mechanism that infants most often exhibit indications for remedies that are considered to have emotional aetiologies – ones such as Lycopodium, Natrum Muriaticum and Sepia – remedies that have 'adult's problems'. It is hard to imagine how else an infant could become a 'Lycopodium type' other than by inheriting the state.

In adult eczema the possible emotional aetiologies are manifold and no different to those found in any other disease state. Such aetiologies as 'ailments from grief' can be useful in confirming some of the smaller remedies, as well as suggesting the better known polychrests. Some examples of this are: Petroleum in the rubric 'Ailments from anger' and Clematis and Graphites in the rubric 'Ailments from grief'.

It is a common mistake, where there is a strong aetiology, to restrict one's view to polychrests. Ignatia or Natrum Muriaticum after bereavement are the obvious examples of this. Prescribing routine remedies in situations like grief will often elicit some sort of response but may well not be curative. Precision is very important if you want to avoid just moving symptoms around and changing the picture without making definite progress.

THE MEDICAL BIOGRAPHY

The importance of the medical history in case-taking is another area well known to homoeopaths. In eczema cases it is particularly important because of the frequent need for nosodes and the consequent requirement to understand the miasmatic influences in the case. Remedy selection too, can be aided by this knowledge. For example,

Clematis and Alumina share certain symptoms but are from different miasmatic groups – Clematis being strongly sycotic and Alumina being mainly psoric. Graphites and Mercurius are a similar example in that Graphites is psoric and Mercurius is mainly syphilitic.

The family medical history can help with the prognosis, too. Some of the most difficult cases, and most failures, occur where there is a complex, mixed miasmatic influence. An unremarkable personal and familial medical history is more likely to make for a straightforward case than one with many chronic diseases in the background. This is especially true if the diseases are on both sides of the family and of mixed miasms, for example, heart disease and arthritis on one side and asthma, cancer and psoriasis on the other. It is a way, therefore, of clarifying both the practitioner's and the patient's expectations.

During the course of treatment the patient may experience new symptoms of various kinds. It is important to know whether they are a return of old symptoms or are truly new for the patient, as this has a bearing on how they are to be assessed and managed. A detailed medical history will help to understand the patient's susceptibilities and alert the practitioner to the likelihood of a previously unresolved or suppressed condition returning, once the healing process is underway.

GENERAL CASE-TAKING TECHNIQUES

It is worth mentioning some of the most useful aspects of case-taking which help us in the understanding of any patient – not just ones with skin complaints. Paragraphs 83 to 99 of the *Organon* give a clear description of case-taking procedure and should be studied thoroughly.

The approach that I have found to be most successful involves putting a structure to the case notes. This is a personal preference and may not suit everyone. Structure leads to simplicity. The information we receive from patients can be distributed into the following categories:

- Details of the chief complaint/s
- Aetiology
- Emotional and mental characteristics – the person behind the symptoms
- Physical generals
- Miasmatic influences – personal and family medical history
- Themes and patterns that run through more than one of the above categories.

Divided up in this way, there are six clearly defined groups of information from which to select prescribing symptoms. If the information in each category is distilled down to what is striking and reliable, the result is a simple yet solid symptom matrix that can lead to a small group of remedies. This is dealt with in detail in Chapter 3.

Some people prefer to work with less rigid structures. 'Mind Maps' as created by Tony Buzan, memory expert and author of *The Mind Map Book* (BBC Publications, 1993), are an example of a more fluid, three-dimensional approach to recording information. Whatever system is adopted, it is important that it should provide quick access and easy recognition of the most important aspects of the case.

Individualise Your Approach

In homoeopathy we pride ourselves in the individual approach we take to treating people and diseases. This emphasis on individualisation should not be restricted to the therapeutics but should begin as soon as we begin to relate to the patient. There can therefore be no one way to take the case; every person has to be approached in a way that will most effectively facilitate the information gathering process in that situation. It requires chameleon-like adaptability on the practitioner's part.

There are patients who can be left to tell their story with little or no interruption, which is all that is required in some circumstances. The concept of 'the minimum dose' is reflected here – the minimum amount of stimulus required to provoke a satisfactory response is always the ideal, in every area of our work. However, in case-taking this does not always work, and there are various reasons why it can be more difficult than that. Some people are not used to talking about themselves in-depth; some do not understand the importance of telling us everything about themselves; some are very reserved or shy and others simply do not have very much to tell. Periods of silence are a well known device to allow the patient to access deep emotions. The skill of waiting is one that applies in many areas of our work and not least in case-taking. However, silence can also be used in an abusive way, sometimes being perceived as threatening or oppressive by the patient. Like everything in homoeopathy, it is not a specific, a universal tool to be used in all situations.

The other extreme to reserve is loquacity, which needs another approach – tactfully guiding the patient back on track and guarding against being drawn into taking down superfluous information that will later confuse the case analysis.

It should also be noted that useful information can come not only from the content of the patient's words but also from the way they express themselves. Loquacity is an obvious symptom that no competent homoeopath would miss. However, symptoms such as 'reserved', 'timidity', 'unobserving' and 'abrupt' can be used where these qualities are marked in the way the patient communicates. There is a section in the repertory – 'Answers' – with many sub-rubrics, that can be helpful. Some examples are:

MIND; ANSWERS; hastily
MIND; ANSWERS; incorrectly
MIND; ANSWERS; irrelevantly
MIND; ANSWERS; monosyllabic
MIND; ANSWERS; slowly

The 'Speech' rubrics should also be referred to. These rubrics describe the quality of the patient's expression and can help to confirm not only polychrests, but some of the 'skin remedies' too. For example, Mezereum has 'Speech, slow' and Dulcamara has 'Speech, stammering'. This is the sort of information that comes only from a combination of observant case-taking and diligent use of the repertory.

In each of the stages of life and in various other situations there are strategies that can aid the case-taking process. I will describe some of the different situations we are confronted with and some ways of approaching them.

Infants and Toddlers

Physical and developmental characteristics should be noted. One of the lessons to be learned here, however, is not to think too stereotypically. Some of the physical signs that can help one to understand the constitution of the child are:

- Tuberculinum babies can be born with a lot of hair on their heads and they will often start walking at an unusually young age, for example 8–10 months. They can also have hair along the spine.
- Babies with very hairy bodies often need Medorrhinum or Thuja.
- Caucasian redheads are very often Phosphorus or Sulphur constitutional types.
- The children that are slow to begin walking are not always Calcarea Carbonica types; the *Complete Repertory* lists 20 remedies in that rubric. 'Slow learning to talk' is another rubric that should be referred to, listing 22 remedies.

31

- Difficult teething is another characteristic that may bias an in-experienced practitioner towards the Calcareas. The *Complete Repertory* lists 74 remedies in the rubric 'Difficult dentition'.
- Babies that have trouble-free dentition are often Phosphorus types. It is the constitutional type that suffers least during teething.
- A large head can be characteristic of Calcarea Carbonica, Calcarea Phosphorica, Silicea and Sulphur. Calcarea Carbonica babies often have a round face and rolls of fat on the neck.
- Caucasian Sulphur babies will often have a ruddy complexion. Sulphur types, despite being warm-blooded, often do not perspire much except at the occiput. They are almost always noticeably warm-blooded and may have a habit of removing their socks.
- Calcarea Carbonica and Phosphorus babies tend to wake cheerful, whereas Lycopodium, Sulphur and Tuberculinum babies are more likely to be irritable on waking.
- Recurrent conjunctivitis with green discharge, also constriction of the prepuce and vaginitis in infants, are signs for Medorrhinum.
- Hair that tangles easily and sticks up at the back of the head is a sign suggesting all the nosodes as well as Mezereum.

Something which may normally be a common symptom, of little use in an adult case, can be helpful in a case with little substance, like that of the infant. For example, in the repertory there is a rubric 'Constipation in children'. A tendency to loose stool is going to be helpful if you are trying to differentiate between Alumina and Sulphur in a case where not many other characteristic symptoms are available. With infants we are dealing with simpler, more general descriptions of things than in adults' cases. Thus 'placid' or 'restless' have more significance than later on in life, when we are able to analyse behaviour in a deeper way. Similarly, a tendency to be nervous or fearless, dependent or independent, will help to eliminate a whole group of remedies, even without being more specific about the exact nature of the behaviour.

If there is one strong characteristic like anxiety or fear of being alone, with no other differentiating symptoms, it can be very helpful to know the mother's case in detail. If, for example, you knew that the mother was an Arsenicum type, the chances of the child responding well to Arsenicum are very good.

Food desires and aversions are extremely useful in children. Our modern repertories have elaborate food sections and a combination like 'averse to sweets and desires fish' can be all you need to arrive at a successful prescription (Phosphorus). The foods I always like to know

32

about are eggs, fish, meat, vegetables, fruit, milk, sweets, salt and spicy. It is surprising how early on in life, for example, a Sulphur child will show a liking for strong-tasting things or how Phosphorus and Sulphur infants prefer savoury baby foods to sweet ones – a useful symptom, since the reverse is usually true in children.

We rely very much on parents for descriptions of their children but this is not always forthcoming in the detail we would like. The information can also come over in a biased way: some parents find it difficult to see any imperfections in their children. Others will stress things that are common for the age group – it is not very often appropriate, for example, to use the symptom 'intolerant of contradiction' in a two- to three-year-old. At least 80% of mothers will describe their toddler as being stubborn. The rubric 'Obstinacy in children' is only reliable if it is a very marked symptom.

Adolescents

This can be one of the most difficult age groups. A co-operative, open adolescent can be a pleasure to work with but all too often they have been brought reluctantly by their parents, or are at the stage of asserting their independence in, perhaps, a quietly defiant way that makes communication difficult. Questions are often answered defensively. It is particularly important to make such patients feel that you are on their side and that the questions are not judgemental in any way. Always suggest seeing them on their own. Some practitioners insist that it is always necessary to spend some time with children without the presence of the parent. I differ in that I feel that even here we have to individualise – some children find this uncomfortable and confrontational, especially during the early stages of their relationship with the practitioner. Always be sensitive to the needs of the patient. It is still necessary to have the views of the parent at this age because many adolescents are only just beginning to become aware of themselves and are not adept at self-examination.

It is helpful with teenagers to demonstrate that you share something in common with them or can relate to them on their level. To show a knowledge of rock music, for example, with someone who has a particular interest in it can help put them at ease, especially if their interest in it is frowned upon at home. Beginning by talking about football or their favourite interest is often better than starting off with probing personal questions.

It is at this age that two behavioural characteristics, interpreted into repertory language, become relevant in the analysis of the case. The symptoms 'reserved' and 'aversion to answer' should not be seen merely as frustrating impediments but also as part of the pathology, if they are very marked.

The treatment of acne in adolescents can be particularly difficult. One of the reasons it is difficult to treat is because of the difficulty in getting to know the patient.

Obtaining a Character Profile

As with the gathering of data about the skin symptoms, it is best to begin with general, open questions and later move on to particulars. There are two basic ways of doing this.

The first is suited to patients who have a knowledge of the homoeo-pathic process or psychosomatic medicine, or who have undergone psychotherapy. Here you can often be almost totally passive and ask the patient to just 'tell their story'. This is the method favoured by many modern classical homoeopaths. The biggest pitfall in these cases is theorising and self-delusion – both on the patient's and the practi-tioner's part. You may also find you are being given too much superfluous information about the person's life, or experiences in a particular area which may not be very relevant to the homoeopathic analysis of the case. Beware of ending the session with pages of psychoanalysis and a dearth of solid, usable facts. Be cautious about taking at face value statements such as 'My problems are all to do with abandonment' from patients who have had a lot of psychotherapy. Sometimes such things are based more on intellectual analysis and theorising than feeling and emotional experience.

The second way is more directive. Begin by simply asking the patient to describe himself or herself. Even if you only get one or two short sentences it can be a very useful way to begin understanding the person. It is common for people to give a list of one-word descriptions like shy, laid-back, placid, tolerant and so on. Such a concise list can reveal several things. The practitioner should at some point go back and try and expand on each of the descriptions and find out more precisely what the patient meant. It is important, though, to get the spontaneous list first – these few words can be the seeds of much deeper insight if they are individually examined. Always be aware that these simple descriptions can say much about the hidden aspects of the person. The number of times patients with suppressed anger have described themselves as placid are too many to number. Never take things on their face value. 'Caring' may mean being in the position of a carer rather than a natural tendency. 'Confident' may relate to the position they have arrived at after years of experience in a profession, but not to social interaction outside that context. Contradictions should be carefully investigated. An example of this was the patient who started by describing herself as lacking confidence and later when asked if she had any fears she replied, 'No, I am a bold person'. That seeming contradiction was a doorway into understanding the patient's emotional make-up in a detailed way.

Always be intent on finding the person behind the symptoms and the individual behind the elementary description.

Some of the other revealing questions to ask are:

- How do others criticise you or complain about you?
- What qualities do you least like in others?
- What qualities do you most admire in others?
- What would you most like to change about yourself?
- How would your wife/husband/partner etc. like you to be different?
- How would you like your present situation to be different?
- How do you like to spend your free time?
- What sort of daydreams or fantasies do you have?
- Tell me more about your relationship with your work colleagues/partner/children/friends.

Avoid asking questions that can be answered by Yes or No. Direct questions should be reserved until the end of the session, to fill in the gaps in your understanding of the patient and for the purpose of remedy differentiation.

People who are totally unable to describe themselves, who seem to have no introspective ability, can be described by the rubric 'un-observing' which is not the same as 'absent-minded', as has been suggested in some repertories.

Just as Hahnemann directs us in the *Organon*, it is helpful to get an impression of the patient from friends and relatives wherever possible.

Symbolic Language

One of the most fascinating aspects of case-taking is the analysis of the patient's use of language. There is much hidden meaning in the words that people subconsciously choose to express themselves. The point is not directly relevant to eczema, but is covered in the case analysis chapter as it is such an important and fascinating subject. This is the main reason why the verbatim recording of patients' words is so valuable. It is not essential; some of the greatest homoeopaths succeed by recording brief descriptions of the patient's symptoms. Some even interpret their words into rubrics as they go along, and with skill and precise application this can work. Verbatim recording does, however, offer us the opportunity to interpret information in a deeper and more creative way. An example of this is the patient who throughout his session used words like 'stagnant', 'stuck' or 'blocked' to describe his physical symptoms. The image was clearly of a person in a very suppressed state, and this was reflected in every aspect of his life right down to the physical sensations associated with his chief complaint. Seeing this theme so clearly helped to select a remedy that suited that type of energetic state.

Questionnaires

These have their pros and cons. If a questionnaire is used, say, to treat patients from a distance, it should be detailed and the questions similar to those posed above. It is surprising how some very reticent or shy patients are able to supply immensely detailed information in a questionnaire. It is worth devising one for the use in difficult situations where you are short of useful information. They can, of course, never replace the consultation as a complete means of case-taking, because the observation aspect of the process is so important. Questionnaires require a lot of patience to fill in properly, too. The one I use in my own practice is 24 pages long and takes about two hours to complete.

Computer Databases

Databases designed specifically for the recording and storing of patient's notes are available. They can be an invaluable tool, allowing access and analysis of our files in a way that would not be possible manually. Any number of variables can be combined and analysed. For example, in a matter of seconds it would be possible to tell how many of your patients in a particular age group have responded to a certain remedy in a specific potency; or how many patients have been referred by a particular doctor and for what condition, and how many of those patients have had successful outcomes. The possibilities are endless. This type of rapid access to large quantities of information will enable us to do important audits of homoeopathic practice. The use of computers for repertorisation, rather than simply for record-keeping or audit, is discussed in the following chapter.

Chapter 3

Case Analysis

REPERTORIES

The techniques of case analysis described in this book are based on the use of the repertory and require a good knowledge of it. Repertories have come a long way since Kent's *Repertory*. While most of the modern repertories use Kent as a basis, they have many additions – both in the rubrics and in the remedies contained in the original rubrics.

To be a consistently effective practitioner without the use of a repertory would require a knowledge of materia medica so vast as to be beyond the capability of anyone not possessing a photographic memory. Some practitioners choose to prescribe intuitively, without referring to the repertory; such an approach is outside the scope of this book.

The repertory is sometimes used to do what can be called 'thumbnail repertorisations', where the content of a rubric or group of rubrics is surveyed visually while analysing the case, either during or after the case-taking session. This can bring to the attention remedies that are running through the symptoms in question and in particular highlight small remedies that are not within the bounds of the practitioner's knowledge of materia medica. It can also be used to confirm suspicions arising out of materia medica knowledge. A case in point would be where Mezereum seems to be well indicated and the patient has a strong desire for coffee and aversion to milk. Referring to those two rubrics could help to confirm the choice of that remedy.

This type of repertory use has its limitations and can also be misleading. It can support incorrect thinking along the lines of an inappropriate remedy.

The most important and useful way of using the repertory is the precise repertorisation of a carefully selected group of symptoms.

37

Precision

Total precision in prescribing is something that we should always aspire to, however difficult it may be. Repertories both assist and limit the sharpness of our precision. To select five rubrics and find that only one relatively unknown remedy runs through those rubrics is very satisfying, if it proves in fact to be the simillimum. It is one of the strengths of the repertory that it can be an essential tool in the solving of that kind of case. These analyses are however relatively rare. Disregarding the various types of practitioner error, there are two main reasons for this with regard to the repertory.

The original Kent's *Repertory* is incomplete in many places. Look for example at the rubrics 'Fastidious', 'Irritability before menses', 'Desires highly seasoned food'. They are clearly incomplete in the number of remedies they contain, and repertorisations will therefore rarely be precise – they will have 'holes' despite the rigour with which rubrics are selected. Using the three rubrics above as an example, Natrum Muriaticum, Pulsatilla, and Sulphur appear in all of them in the *Complete Repertory* but would barely feature using Kent's *Repertory*. Nosodes are poorly represented in Kent, indeed some do not feature at all, so an important part of our therapeutic arsenal is put further out of our reach than we would wish. Until recently it was not possible to find an indicated nosode, other than Psorinum, by precise repertorisation.

Larger and more modern books present us with a different problem in relation to our attempt to be precise. It is common with such repertories, because of the number of additions to them, to arrive at a group of ten or more remedies rather than one or two. As the repertories and rubrics get bigger, the way we use them will have to adapt. Often the most that a repertory can do for you is lead you to a relatively large group of remedies amongst which you will hopefully find the simillimum. To a certain extent that has always been the case, but the difference now is that the group of remedies arrived at is getting bigger. This can work both for and against you. It may make you aware of important remedies you might otherwise have overlooked, or it might confuse with too many choices.

The main aim of this book is to improve the precision of prescribing by distilling our knowledge down to what is most useful in practice. Although seminar presentations and articles in journals often portray examples of extraordinarily precise prescribing, day-to-day practice is not always like that. Elegant precision is an exception rather than the rule, even in the best homoeopathic practice.

Computers

Repertorisation is a task perfectly suited to computers, since it involves time-consuming and tedious calculation. Once a computer has been used in daily practice for some time it is difficult to imagine ever having coped without one.

Computer repertories offer several analysis options. The one favoured in this book is the 'number of rubrics' analysis. In other words, no weight is given to the grading of the symptoms or of the remedies in the rubrics. This is because the aim is to repertorise only what is characteristic of the case and to try to select symptoms that are reliable. A repertory chart generated by a computer is a list of the possible indicated remedies and a useful graphic representation of your reasons for prescribing. Even if the prescribed remedy was not arrived at by repertorisation, the repertory graph will serve as a summary of the characteristic symptoms of the case for future use. For this second reason it is worth repertorising every case, even if the prescription is arrived at by means other than the repertory.

Some computer programmes have facilities like 'expert systems', whose use requires that symptoms are graded in importance or intensity. An expert system not only repertorises but also analyses the case, being modelled on the thought processes of a homoeopath – in other words an attempt to make the computer 'think' like a practitioner. These computer programmes can no doubt be very useful, but are outside the scope of this work.

Repeated use of the repertory is one of the best ways of learning materia medica without really trying. After years of looking at rubrics many times over, their contents begin to stick in the mind. Eventually the remedies in common rubrics such as 'Forsaken feeling', 'Desires salt or salty food', or 'Itching worse at night' are recalled through familiarity with those rubrics.

Specific remedies can be studied in the repertory, too, and this method has been used by many teachers for a long time. However, trawling through the printed version of a repertory in search of the occurrences of a remedy is a laborious task, and the same can be achieved in seconds by the search facility of a computer repertory. Thus one can find all the delusions of Kali Bromatum, or the food desires and aversions of Physostigma, or all the grade 3 occurrences of a remedy in a particular section of the repertory. The examples are endless.

As with most things, computers have their drawbacks, and over-reliance on them can lead to wrong prescriptions. Because repertorisation is so simplified by the computer, it is possible to make the error of putting too many symptoms into the repertorisation – ending up with an abundance of polychrests and quite possibly wrong remedies in the analysis. There are pitfalls even when carefully selecting smaller numbers of rubrics.

The temptation is to prescribe remedies that would not normally be considered for a case just because they have scored highly in the repertorisation. The computer can remind you of remedies you might have overlooked but equally suggest remedies that are totally inappropriate. It is one of the characteristics of repertorisation that even well-selected rubrics can bring out inappropriate remedies at times, and it is often difficult to be sure if the computer is revealing a facet of a remedy that you are not aware of. This is more likely to happen if your attention is focused on the computer screen rather than on the person sitting in front of you. One of the fundamentals of repertorisation is always to refer back to the materia medica to select the simillimum from the list of possible remedies suggested by the repertory.

PARTICULARS IN CASE ANALYSIS

In the treatment of eczema, particulars – especially the symptoms of the skin – can be very useful. One of the most important aims of this chapter is to develop and clarify the following point: *The level on which characteristic symptoms express themselves, and the extent to which particular symptoms are relevant in the analysis, vary from case to case and mostly according to the degree of pathology present.*

With the development of modern psychologically-oriented homoeopathy, much emphasis has been put on understanding 'the person behind the symptoms'. Homoeopaths agree that most disease is not a local affection and that the disease process is as complex as the person manifesting the symptoms – that is, it is a product of the patient's total state of being. However, the accepted hierarchy of symptoms, in which mental and emotional symptoms take precedence over physical ones, is not always appropriate in eczema. There is nothing wrong with that model *per se*, but it does not fit every type of case. In particular, it cannot work if there is a paucity of mental and emotional symptoms. As will be shown, that is often the scenario with which one is confronted in the treatment of eczema cases.

Our knowledge of the injurious effects of suppressing eruptions with allopathic medicines, together with the tendency – usually quite correctly – to avoid prescribing on the basis of superficial physical symptoms, has given rise to some misunderstanding of the homoeo-pathic treatment of eczema. As a result, many patients receive disappointing treatment and many homoeopaths proclaim that skin problems are very difficult to treat, perhaps, in some cases, developing philosophical excuses for failure. Misplaced fear of suppression with homoeopathy can lead to practitioner confusion and inaccurately prescribed remedies. That is not to say that we should cease to be mindful of the possibility of suppression; hopefully this chapter will help to clarify the point.

Symptoms are important to the extent to which they characterise or individualise a case. Characteristic symptoms can manifest on any level. The fact that the eruption itches more at night is as much characteristic of the 'state of disposition' (*Organon*, Paragraph 211) as any other aspect of the case. We should not be put off by the fact that the symptom is physical or that it is a skin symptom. There is a lot of mythology surrounding the evils of 'treating the skin', as if the skin is somehow separate from the rest of the person and not part of the totality. There is a belief that it can be suppressive to use skin symptoms in the analysis of the case, and that it is more important to understand the mentals and generals than the particulars. As is so often the case in homoeopathy, the latter is *often* but not *always* true. Unfortunately, guidelines may mistakenly become rules, and the important exceptions to what is common get overlooked at a cost to our patients. It has been said that the one word which answers every question that can be asked about homoeopathy is 'Sometimes'!

There is a spectrum of possibilities beginning at the point where particulars – because they are common symptoms – are useless, through to the other extreme where the particular symptoms are the totality and there is nothing else to go on – no individualising mental or general symptoms. There are clearly many degrees in between these two extremes.

In his book *The Spirit of Homoeopathy*, Rajan Sankaran states: 'A remedy that covers the mental state and general symptoms of a patient has got a greater possibility of curing than the one that covers the par-ticulars without covering the mentals and generals.' This is true, *as long as there are individualising mentals and generals with which to work.*

It should be remembered that the skin has important sensory, neurological, eliminative, thermostatic and other functions, and that even in physiological terms it tells us much about the inner condition of the person. In homoeopathic terms, the skin can be equally important in the way it can reveal useful aspects of the totality of symptoms.

WHICH TOTALITY?

'The pathological manifestations accessible to our senses express all the internal changes, i.e., the whole pathological disturbance of the dynamis: they reveal the whole disease.' (*Organon*, Paragraph 12)

'The 'totality of symptoms' means a good deal. It is a wonderfully broad thing. It may be considered to be all that is essential of the disease.' (*Lectures on Homoeopathic Philosophy*, J.T. Kent)

Where does the totality of symptoms begin and end? Does it stop just below the patient's skin? On the surface of the skin? Does it extend beyond the skin into the patient's personal world? Is the patient's environment the cause of the totality or part of the totality?

It is my view that the real totality has no boundary. Our understanding of the totality is determined only by our ability to perceive it. Thus Hahnemann uses the phrase in Paragraph 12: '...manifestations accessible to our senses...' It is possible that in the future we will be able to diagnose the simillimum on a microscopic level. It is certain that the individuality of the patient and his or her disease can reveal itself on that level, but as yet we do not have the ability to interpret it. The modern technique of dark-field microscopy of live blood reveals a living, unique picture of the person. Surely the essence of the person is expressed as much in that myriad of life forms and biological relationships as it is in the way we relate to the outside world.

An alternative view is that our understanding is determined by how much of the totality the organism chooses to reveal to us at any one time. Either way, the clues we use to understand the case may exist on any one of a multitude of levels. We may use a small group of physical generals and particulars, or we may take into consideration the patient's childhood, the state of the mother during pregnancy, the nature of their personal relationships, or maybe even, taking the broadest view, the type of problems they are currently having with their car or any other inanimate object with which they are intimately associated!

It is best to approach every case with the intention of perceiving the largest possible totality. We can then scale down our view and refocus, until we are able to perceive what is to be cured in the individual. We allow the patient and their symptoms to determine the approach we are to use rather than beginning with a preconceived methodology. A practitioner who can see a large totality can choose to prescribe on a small one when the clinical situation demands it, but the prescriber who sees only the small totality is unable to do the reverse.

THE HOLOGRAM ANALOGY

The way we view our patient and analyse their homoeopathic case can be compared to the characteristics, and our perception of, holograms.

In simple terms, a hologram, or three-dimensional image of light, is made in the following way:

A laser beam is passed through a device called a beam splitter, which creates a reference beam and an object beam out of the original beam of light. The object beam is directed at the object of which the holographic image is to be made and another laser is passed through the interference pattern created by the combination of the reflected object and reference beams. The result is a three-dimensional image of the object.

Holograms have some extraordinary characteristics. Take a small part of the hologram, pass another laser through it and the whole of the original image is reproduced. Each time this is done, the original object is duplicated, but from a different perspective, no matter how many such sub–images are created. The whole is contained within the tiniest part. This same phenomenon is seen in fractal geometry, in which an organised structure is found to be hidden within complex shapes. (The book *Chaos* by James Gleick (Cardinal, 1990) is an excellent introduction to fractals and the concept of self-similarity – patterns within patterns that repeat themselves to infinity.) The geometrical pattern of an image such as the Mandelbrot Set or the Koch Curve is repeated over and over, however small a part of the original image you observe.

In the case of holograms, the smaller the piece you take to make your new image, the less clearly defined that new image will be. The more the process is repeated, the less clear the image becomes. But the more individual images you take – because each is from a different perspective – the clearer you will be about what you are looking at.

Correspondences with the Homoeopathic Case

The above characteristics of the hologram are analogous to the homoeopathic perception of the case:

1) The whole is present in the tiniest part. The small group of characteristic symptoms contain the essence of the whole case. Say for example, an eczema case that has the following features:

   SKIN; ERUPTIONS; fissured
   SKIN; ERUPTIONS; winter; agg.
   SKIN; ITCHING; scratching; changing place, on
   SKIN; ITCHING; warm, becoming

This matrix of symptoms is unique to Alumina (using *The Complete Repertory*). Providing these symptoms are reliable, i.e. in frequency and intensity, Alumina can be prescribed with reasonable confidence (providing also that the symptoms are not being used at the expense of characteristic mental and general symptoms and that there are no contraindications for Alumina). The essence of the case is expressing itself in a unique way through these local symptoms. The whole is contained in the part.

2) The smaller the group of symptoms we look at, the less clear the image of the patient/disease. This is analogous to using a very small part of the original hologram to recreate the original image.

   Obviously, the fewer the symptoms, the less use they are on their own. Take the following two symptoms:

SKIN; ERUPTIONS; discharging, moist; scratching, after
SKIN; ITCHING; night

There are eighteen remedies common to those two rubrics.

3) The more 'stepped-down' (a term used to describe an electrical current passed through a transformer in order to reduce the voltage) the symptoms are, the less reliable they will be. This explains that physical particular symptoms on their own are generally less reliable and useful than symptoms of the mind and physical generals. This is especially true if the disturbance has its origin on the emotional level – the skin symptoms are a 'stepped-down' expression of that disturbance.

4) The more small images you look at, the clearer you are about what is to be cured in the patient. The whole will be contained within each part. Therefore it is often the case that the small totality of the skin, the small totality of the digestive system and the bigger totality of the mind will all express the same theme and will reveal a thread that runs through the case, enabling the correct selection of the simillimum. It is usually in this situation that the simillimum is chosen with the greatest accuracy.

Remedies Vary in Size

Similarly, our remedies have varying sizes of totality. That may be because:

- The nature of the substance from which the remedy is made is such that it has an inherently small totality of symptoms. Just as there are simple cases and complex cases, there are simple remedies and complex remedies. It is difficult to say what determines this relative simplicity/complexity. In the case of the mineral remedies it may perhaps be related to the position of the remedy or its components in the Periodic Table. With animal and plant remedies it is possible that an in-depth investigation of the substance in question might answer the question. There is no general rule that can be applied in order to understand this. It is an interesting question to consider why Ignatia, Nux Vomica and Pulsatilla have such bigger, more elaborate pictures than say, Asparagus, Prunus Spinosa and Symphytum.

- We may not have yet brought out the full totality by a thorough proving or by clinical experience and frequent use of the remedy. Modern homoeopathy has understood, and continues to develop many so-called small remedies in a deeper and broader way. This is happening all the time at a great rate. This is largely due to our modern understanding of the emotions and psychosomatism, as well as present-day homoeopaths' desire to understand the whole materia medica in a more profound way rather than relying on keynotes alone.

It is, for example, adequate to know that Benzoic Acid has urine that smells like horse's urine and is brown in colour, that there is an amelioration when sediment is passed and that it has an affinity for the heart and gouty joint problems. It is, however, more helpful to know that the remedy can also have hypochondriasis, desire to be carried and dwelling on past disagreeable occurrences. To be able to take it a stage further back, and understand the situation in which the Benzoic Acid state tends to develop, would be even more helpful.

It is an important service to homoeopathy to develop remedies in this way. Each time you *successfully* use a small remedy, exploit the situation as much as possible in order to understand the remedy as fully as you can. By comparing these findings with other cured cases the materia medica can become more complete.

Our relationship with the materia medica should be the same as that with our patients. We should never be content to take things at face value or understand things in a superficial way. Our aim should always be to perceive the 'bigger picture' and comprehend the totality in a holistic way.

CHARACTERISTIC SYMPTOMS

It is not possible to be consistently effective as a homoeopath if you are rigid in your approach to case analysis. If you believe that every case can be solved by analysing the mind alone, or by prescribing on the skin symptoms alone, you will have many disappointments. In the 1980s and 1990s homoeopathy has gone through a wonderful renaissance in which its psychological element has predominated. It may also have become a little unbalanced that way. We see many good cases presented in journals and at seminars that demonstrate psychological homoeopathy. Terms such as 'central delusion', around which the whole case revolves, are common. Some teachers go as far as describing the individual's state of health as their conflict with God. More and more elaborate remedy essences are being developed. This type of homoeopathy is in a way most inspiring and interesting – an approach that seeks to understand the patient's place in the universe, relate their symptoms to it, and interpret that understanding into homoeopathic sense.

Many cases in day-to-day practice, however, are not of that nature and require a different approach. It is an essential skill to be able to know from where, amongst the vast, or maybe scanty, amount of information received from the patient, to select your prescribing symptoms.

It is interesting that Hahnemann, in the *Organon*, Paragraph 153, directs us only to find 'the more striking, strange, unusual and peculiar (characteristic) signs and symptoms in the case'. Nowhere does he state that only mental symptoms should be used, or that they always more important than physical symptoms.

It can be difficult to discern what is useful in a case and what is not. At which level should treatment be aimed? To a certain extent the answer to this question should be obvious. Provided the case is taken properly, the case analysis should 'solve itself'. The useful information in a case is what is left over after you have discarded what is useless! There are several aspects to defining the relative usefulness of information.

1) Choose the 'more striking, strange, unusual, peculiar (characteristic) symptoms in the case' (*Organon*, Paragraph 153). These symptoms can occur on the mental, emotional or physical level. Symptoms can be characteristic in several ways:

   i) In terms of their permanence, regularity and intensity. If a patient mentions the symptom of a sensation of a mouse running across their skin, there is no doubt that this is strange, rare and peculiar, but it will be vastly more important if it is a frequent recurrence than if it has only happened once. Similarly, an itch that is worse from warmth 'sometimes' is a lot less reliable than one for whom warmth is intolerable.

A judgement has to be made as to whether the symptom is out of proportion to the circumstances. This especially applies to mental symptoms. To take a simple example: most people have fear of heights standing on the edge of a cliff, whereas a terror of climbing a two-metre ladder would be out of proportion.

If a symptom is either part of a repeating pattern or reflects a theme in the patient's life, it is of the highest order of importance and reliability. So 'Ailments from disappointed love', for example, would be more essential to the core of the analysis if it was a repeating pattern than if it was a one-off event. Similarly, if we deduce that the theme in the patient's life is 'changeability' or 'ungroundedness', the symptoms 'itch, wandering' becomes important in that it is symbolic of the general state of the person. It is also a way of expressing the state of the patient without 'trying too hard' to find an appropriate mental or general rubric to express the idea, and in doing so, to run the risk of choosing a misleading one. Homoeopaths who have a background in Chinese medicine and the Five Elements are able to make even more sense of the inter-relationship of symptoms in this way.

ii) Symptoms can be peculiar in their own right. For example, a sensation as if the skin is hanging loose (Belladonna, Kreosotum, Phosphorus, Sabadilla) or yellow discolouration in circles (Natrum Carbonicum).

iii) Symptoms can be peculiar if they are unusual for the disease. For example, itching that is better for warmth, or an eruption that is concomitant with diarrhoea.

iv) Symptoms can be peculiar to a small number of remedies. For example, eruptions on uncovered parts (Thuja) or itching that is worse for washing in cold water (Clematis).

v) A definite aetiology can be a characteristic symptom. For example, eczema since vaccination, emotional upset, acute illness, etc.

vi) Any symptoms with marked modalities are important characteristic symptoms.

2) Knowledge of the repertory adds another dimension to selecting symptoms. Knowing that a particular rubric is either too large to be useful or too small to be reliable will help us to include or discard symptoms. For example, the sensation of bubbling on the skin is unusual but the repertory only lists one remedy (Calcarea Carbonica), so this symptom is unlikely to help us much except as a confirmatory symptom where everything else is pointing to Calcarea Carbonica. On the other hand, the patient may experience very severe forgetfulness, but knowing that there are about two hundred remedies listed with that symptom will help us to de-emphasise it as a prescribing symptom. There is an obvious correlation between largeness of rubrics and commonness of symptoms. There are however a few exception to this, for example the rubrics:

MIND; CHEERFULNESS – 226 remedies
MIND; DISCONTENTED – 183 remedies
MIND; DISCOURAGED – 142 remedies
MIND; MALICIOUS – 96 remedies
SKIN; ERYSIPELAS – 127 remedies

It may be that one of the most characteristic symptoms in the case is the tendency to become very easily discouraged. This is not a common symptom, but the rubric will be of little use because of its size. Our knowledge of materia medica can of course make such information more useful. We know, for example, that Baryta Carbonica and Graphites are more likely to experience feeling easily discouraged than Causticum or Ferrum.

On the other hand, a fairly common symptom may have a surprisingly small rubric, for example:

MIND; ENVY – 21 remedies
SKIN; ITCHING; wool; agg. – 11 remedies
GENERALITIES; TOBACCO; desires; smoking – 16 remedies

These guidelines may seem simplistic, but it is precisely by applying simple criteria of this kind to your analysis strategy that your cases will be helped to 'solve themselves'.

Always remember to try and perceive the biggest possible totality while at the same time not overlooking the small details of the symptoms of the skin.

LACK OF MENTAL SYMPTOMS

Skin symptoms should not be given precedence over, or used at the expense of, characteristic mental and general symptoms. However, many homoeopaths are likely to agree that eczema patients often present with very few useful mental symptoms. There are of course many exceptions, and there exist many purely psychosomatic eczema cases which are treated in the conventional classical way. However, compared to any other common complaint (perhaps other than osteoarthritis), there is a large proportion of one-sided cases with few core emotional symptoms. Many eczema patients appear relatively well balanced or with little to say of an existential nature.

There is a possible reason for this. *A relatively healthy organism will manifest its disturbance on the surface – on the skin – as far away from vital organs and the mental and emotional levels as possible.* Therefore, it stands to reason that a 'healthy' person, one with good vitality and who is emotionally well balanced, is more likely to present with skin problems than inner functional disorders or pathology. Similarly, an organism that has managed to manifest its disturbance on the skin is less likely to have mental or emotional symptoms as a direct result of having done so. It appears to be a straightforward example of Hering's Law of Cure in action, and follows Hahnemann's theory of chronic disease.

ACORNS AND OAKS

Let us look at the disease process in analogous terms. The analogy of the germinating seed maturing into a fully grown plant mirrors the stages of development in chronic disease. It offers a helpful way of clarifying the concept of layers and the relevance of particulars in case analysis.

When the seed of a plant begins to germinate, the first sprout that appears above the soil is unrecognisable as a particular plant. It is characterless. It goes without saying that the more expert the observer, the greater the possibility of early identification. As the plant grows it begins to take a shape. After a while it will become clear whether the plant is, say, a tree, a grass or a root vegetable. There will be an intermediate stage when the identity of the plant will still be indeterminate. It may be clear that it is not a type of grass, but whether it is an oak, an elm or a birch will be difficult to tell. The next stage is adulthood, when even to the untrained observer it is quite obvious what sort of plant it is. It has a definite character, a shape, colour and character. The plant may grow to the point of overwhelming the container that holds it – the pot in which the seed was planted becomes totally obscured by the foliage.

In homoeopathic terms, the disease process goes through the following similar stages.

The early stages of chronic disease reveal little that is characteristic and usable in the analysis, and we have to rely on mental and general symptoms. We treat the 'container' and the 'soil' rather than the plant (the outer manifestation of the disease process). At this stage the 'plant' is unrecognisable and it is not even certain that it will survive. As with the plant however, the more expert the observer, the greater the likelihood of identification. An experienced homoeopath needs less information than a novice upon which to base a prescription.

As the disease develops, it begins to develop a semblance of character. Modalities appear. We are now able to include some of the symptoms of the disease in the analysis.

Once the disease reaches its full expression, it will be rich in symptoms. We will be presented with sensation, location, extension and modalities. Another level of information may become available as the language that the patient uses to describe the complaint becomes more elaborate. The analysis at this stage may include elements from every level – mental, emotional, physical generals and particulars.

The final – overwhelming – stage is when 'the person behind the disease' is obscured. The symptoms of the disease have become uppermost. In these cases there will be few mental or general symptoms unless they are very much part of the disease picture. It is here that smaller remedies are called for – remedies with narrow spheres of action and with a small number of characteristic symptoms; in the case of eczema these will usually, but not exclusively, be physical ones. This is discussed in more detail in the chapter on materia medica.

SEVERE CASES AND THE 'SMALL TOTALITY'

Symptom Matrices

The term 'symptom matrix' is used to describe an array of symptoms (usually two to six) which precisely describes a 'small totality' of skin symptoms and which, when repertorised, leads to a small group of remedies.

The skin section of the repertory is particularly rich in useful rubrics, probably more so than sections that cover complaints of the musculo-skeletal, respiratory or digestive systems. There is no particular explanation for this and the observation is based on practical experience.

As has already been discussed, the more severe the complaint, and the fewer the mental and general symptoms, the more the symptoms of the skin become important to the practitioner. There are many symptoms of eczema, some fairly common and others more unusual, that occur in different combinations in individuals. These combinations form unique matrices which, when repertorised, lead you to a group of remedies. Here are a few examples of such matrices:

- SKIN; ERUPTIONS; washing; agg.
  SKIN; ITCHING; night
  SKIN; ITCHING; warm, becoming

  Clematis, Mezereum, Psorinum, Sarsaparilla, Sulphur and Urtica Urens are in all three of these rubrics. Without the use of the repertory, and relying on materia medica knowledge alone, many practitioners would prescribe Sulphur on the basis of these symptoms (in the absence of more information) and possibly overlook a more appropriate remedy.

- SKIN; ITCHING; night
  SKIN; ITCHING; scratch; must; until it bleeds
  SKIN; ITCHING; warm, becoming

  Bovista, Dolichos, Ledum, Mezereum, Psorinum and Pulsatilla appear in this group.

- SKIN; ITCHING; evening
  SKIN; ITCHING; scratch; must; until it is raw
  SKIN; ITCHING; warm, becoming

  Alumina, Lycopodium, Mercurius, Mezereum and Pulsatilla.

These examples show how a subtle difference in the skin symptoms can make a significant change to the group of remedies you are looking at.

Another two examples of matrices:

- SKIN; ERUPTIONS; discharging, moist; scratching, after
  SKIN; ITCHING; night
  SKIN; ITCHING; scratching; amel.
  SKIN; ITCHING; undressing; agg.

  Bovista, Kreosotum, Ledum, Mercurius, Mezereum, Oleander and Sulphur.

- SKIN; ERUPTIONS; discharging, moist; scratching, after
  SKIN; ERUPTIONS; winter; agg.
  SKIN; ITCHING; wool; agg.

  Hepar Sulphuris and Sulphur.

If there are strong 'constitutional' or mental and general indications for a remedy, those indications should be given precedence over local ones. Similarly, if the local symptoms suggest a remedy that is strongly contraindicated by the mental and general symptoms of the patient, it should not be given. *Local symptoms can complement, but should never be used at the expense of, characteristic mental and general symptoms.*

Small Totality Case Examples

This is often a stage at the beginning of treatment while symptoms are still severe. It may also be a phase in the treatment when 'unsuppression' is taking place, as the vital force begins to react against the long-term effects of suppressive treatment and the disease is revealed in its true form. It is the stage where the skin symptoms are uppermost – the final stage of the 'plant analogy'. The plant is fully developed and now overwhelms and obscures the vessel in which it is growing. Such cases were called 'one-sided' by Hahnemann. The remedy used at this time may be the simillimum that takes the patient all the way to a cure, but much more commonly it is one of several remedies that will be needed as the case unfolds. This has been referred to as the zigzag way to cure.

Hahnemann describes the process of treating one-sided diseases in Paragraphs 172–84 of the *Organon*. He advises that the most well indicated remedy should be selected on the basis of the small number of symptoms available. He goes on to explain that sometimes this remedy will cure, especially where the symptoms are striking, uncommon and characteristic (Paragraph 178). However, in most cases, the initial prescription, based on the one-sided disease picture, will reveal new symptoms that can then be used to select a second prescription (Paragraph 180). Hahnemann explains that even though the new symptoms are brought out by the first prescription, they are part of the disease and should be used as such (Paragraph 181).

The best way to illustrate this is by means of examples. All the cases in this book are presented in a summarised form with the purpose of illustrating a particular point. Many are distilled from several pages of notes.

CASE 1

A little boy just over one year old. When he first came for treatment there was very little to go on constitutionally. The whole case was overwhelmed by skin symptoms. The child was really distressed by the eczema, constantly scratching and rubbing at it and very upset and crying most of the time. There was no family history to go on and no clear miasmatic influence on the basis of diseases in the family background. The symptoms were:

SKIN; CRACKS, fissures; deep, bloody
SKIN; ERUPTIONS; discharging, moist; bloody
SKIN; ERUPTIONS; fetid
SKIN; ITCHING; night
SKIN; ITCHING; warm, becoming

The opening remedy on the basis of these symptoms was Mercurius Solubilis. He was put on Mercurius 6c three times a day for a month. When he next came the skin was less cracked and he was calmer in himself. He was kept on the Mercurius 6c. One month later he had improved a little more but his father felt the improvement had slowed down, so the potency was increased to 12c three times a day. One month after that it was increased to Mercurius 30c once a day.

Unfortunately the increase in potency at that stage was premature and he relapsed fairly badly, although he did not go 'back to square one'. The decision to increase the potency at that point, from 12c to 30c, was based more on practitioner impatience than the needs of the patient. He went back to 12c and stayed on that for a further six weeks. At the next visit, which was about four and a half months after starting treatment, the picture had changed. The skin symptoms were much less severe and less characteristic – *the symptoms of the person were beginning to emerge.*

The analysis of the case changed as is the case once improvement has been established with the lesional remedy. The symptoms now selected were:

MIND; FASTIDIOUS. (This was shown by his dislike of dirty hands and face, and unlike most children of his age, he was averse to eating with his hands because of the mess it made. He would also pick fluff off his father's clothes while he held him.)

HEAD; PERSPIRATION; scalp; sleep; during

GENERALITIES; FOOD and drinks; spices, condiments, piquant, highly seasoned food; desires

SKIN; ITCHING; air; cold; agg.

On repertorising these symptoms, the remedy was very clearly Sepia. Sepia follows well after Mercurius, which is an important consideration. These stages or layers do not happen randomly – it is essential always to pay attention to the relationship of remedies in cases like this. It can be a useful guide as to what the next remedy should be. He was given Sepia 12c twice a day.

He progressed on Sepia but after a few weeks regressed slightly with a return of a mild itchy rash. He was given Sulphur for a while as it had also come up in the repertorisation, but with no effect. Sepia was resumed, whereupon he improved again.

The remedy Phosphorus, which follows Sepia well and is complementary to it, completed the treatment. Phosphorus is his constitutional remedy and has proved most effective at keeping him healthy, as well as for treating acute illnesses. At the beginning of treatment the Phosphorus was neither 'visible' nor appropriate.

CASE 2

A little girl with eczema with the following symptoms:

SKIN; ERUPTIONS; vesicular; itching

SKIN; ERUPTIONS; washing; agg.

SKIN; ITCHING; night

SKIN; ITCHING; warm, becoming

It was another example of a case with very few characteristic mentals and generals upon which to prescribe. The only symptoms of use were those of the skin.

The opening prescription was Sulphur, which aggravated the

condition with no subsequent amelioration. The other remedy in all the rubrics was Clematis. Using Clematis over a period of nine months she became eruption-free. Sulphur was needed to finish off the case, with the symptoms:

FACE; DISCOLORATION; red; circumscribed
SKIN; ITCHING; eruption; without
SKIN; ITCHING; night
SKIN; ITCHING; warm, becoming

There was a certain amount of concern about the chances of success with this case as the mother was new to homoeopathy and had more or less been persuaded to come by her neighbour. In situations like these it is rare to have the luxury of time to allow for mistakes. It was therefore particularly gratifying to have a positive outcome, especially as it involved an unusual remedy, which always increases practitioner satisfaction!

Clematis appears to be a remedy that has a relatively small picture and does not much pervade the mental/emotional sphere. It has a few interesting mental symptoms such as 'Ailments from homesickness', 'Fear of being alone with aversion to company' and 'Sensitive to all external impressions', but it will usually be prescribed on the basis of physical symptoms, whether skin symptoms or those of the urinary tract (its other main affinity).

CASE 3

This is a case of a 26-year-old woman who had eczema from birth. Hers was a totally one-sided case with no mental symptoms at all. She was a perfectly happy, well balanced person and did not even have a single general symptom of importance. However her eczema had the following characteristics:

EXTREMITIES; CRACKED skin; hands
SKIN; ERUPTIONS; discharging, moist
SKIN; ERUPTIONS; perspiring parts, on
SKIN; ERUPTIONS; vesicular; small
SKIN; ERUPTIONS; winter; agg.
SKIN; EXCORIATION; scratching, after
SKIN; ITCHING; scratching; amel.

Repertorising these symptoms led to Rhus Toxicodendron, which cleared the condition. There is no other way the simillimum could have been found in this case.

CASE 4

This case demonstrates some important aspects of treating eczema. It was a woman in her fifties with severe eczema all over her body, which had been controlled with cortisone for many years. Her characteristic eczema symptoms were:

SKIN; CRACKS, fissures; deep, bloody
SKIN; ERUPTIONS; suppressed
SKIN; ERUPTIONS; winter; agg.

She had been given a sequence of ineffective remedies by another homoeopath, which helped to narrow down the choice. She was prescribed Petroleum 12c and later 30c daily. As the skin improved it moved down her body until only her lower legs had any eruption. It stopped improving on Petroleum at this point. She telephoned to say that she had been at a friend's house where a dermatologist who was visiting there had seen her legs and told her she should be in hospital, as her legs were septic and ulcerating.

The new symptom matrix was as follows. Once again there were no useful mental or general symptoms:

SKIN; CRACKS; deep, bloody
SKIN; ERUPTIONS; suppurating
SKIN; ULCERS; discharges; green

Mercurius 12c repeated four times a day got her over that stage quickly.

One of the most important aspects of this approach – prescribing on what is uppermost in the case and using skin symptom matrices – is the need for the homoeopath to be very precise in assessing the response to each remedy, and to be vigilant for a change in the centre of gravity of the symptomatology. Often, mental and general symptoms will begin to appear, or gain more significance to the patient, as the symptoms of the skin subside. A child will begin by having a generally poor appetite, say, and later begin to develop likes and dislikes. Mental symptoms will become more usable. For example, fretfulness and sleeplessness might become fastidiousness and sleeplessness between 2 a.m. and 4 a.m.

Some readers may have alarm bells ringing at this point and be considering suppression, with the apparent progression of symptoms from the physical to the mental level. This is an important point. There is a difference between the development of mental pathology, with the disappearance of physical symptoms and the emergence of the constitutional characteristics of the person. Whatever else happens, there should always be an improvement in the general wellbeing of the patient.

The development of totally new symptoms that are limiting to the patient is a sign of suppression. For example, sleeplessness, loss of appetite, irritability, anxiety or tiredness, where such symptoms did not exist before, would be a bad sign. The appearance of a symptom such as fastidiousness, fear of dogs or desire for salt are characteristics of polychrests and common constitutional remedies like Calcarea Carbonica, Phosphorus, Sulphur, etc. Such characteristics will often be obscured or will not manifest at times of severe exacerbation of the skin symptoms, but will become more apparent as the eczema improves and the 'next layer' reveals itself.

There are many exceptions to this, and most of them involve polychrests in which, however intense the physical symptoms, the remedy image can express itself on every level of the organism. One obvious example of this is Sulphur, which will rarely express itself just in a local way – it will usually also manifest some mental and general symptoms. Similarly, a remedy like Arsenicum, with its striking mental symptoms, will rarely manifest physical symptoms alone. A state in which there are intense physical symptoms with marked modalities and no characteristic mental symptoms is most likely to indicate that a small remedy is appropriate.

It is however surprising how often a polychrest will not be evident on the basis of mental symptoms. The following case is one in which physical general and particular symptoms were used to find a remedy which is normally prescribed on the basis of mental symptoms:

CASE 5

This was a little boy who had a strong modality of being worse from heat. Not only was the itch worse but he was totally 'out of sorts' when he got hot, and adored being fanned and felt much better for it. He radiated heat like a little heater. This was the overwhelming characteristic of the case. The rubrics chosen were:

SKIN; ERUPTIONS; bleeding; scratching, after
SKIN; ITCHING; night
GENERALITIES; FANNED; being; amel.
GENERALITIES; HEAT; sensation of
GENERALITIES; HEATED, becoming

The remedy was Lachesis, which took the heat right out of his body. It was like turning off a switch. Again, that was one stage in the treatment and he went on to require other remedies, although nothing would work until he had had the Lachesis – he had been given several remedies before it with no effect. This was surprising, because there was no apparent jealousy in the case and no mental symptoms at all. It is not often that Lachesis is prescribed on physical symptoms alone.

CASE 6

This is another example, with similar symptoms, that demonstrates the same idea:

It is a constant challenge to remain broad-minded enough to allow for the non-obvious in homoeopathic practice. This case made me realise that I had been thinking too much in terms of what, according to my experience, were 'eczema remedies' and 'children's remedies'.

A girl, five years of age, had been having homoeopathic treatment for severe eczema and asthma without success from an experienced practitioner for over a year. It was a very one-sided case. Apart from the fact that she was extremely affectionate and sensitive to admonition, there were not many mental symptoms of use in the case. The eczema was all over the body and very itchy. The itch was worse at night, worse from warmth, and better for being fanned. The child insisted on taking her fan everywhere with her. The asthma was worse in the evening, as regular as clockwork, as soon as the sun went down.

Over a period of two years the child had Sulphur, Pulsatilla, Lachesis, Natrum Muriaticum, Graphites, Sanicula, Carcinosin, Medorrhinum, Tuberculinum, Lycopodium, Psorinum, Thuja and Calcarea Carbonica, with only marginal and temporary improvements in the eczema and no change in the asthma. She also tried a strict elimination diet with no result. Eventually I decided to take the two rubrics that expressed the most constant and reliable symptoms in the case:

RESPIRATION; ASTHMATIC; evening
GENERALITIES; FANNED; desire to be

Besides Pulsatilla and Sulphur, Zincum is the only other remedy in both the rubrics. This remedy over a period of a few months had an unprecedented effect on the asthma and the eczema. China Officinalis completed the cure.

It looks very simple presented this way, but for two years wrong remedies were chosen by being too complicated, i.e. by using too many symptoms and looking for mental symptoms where there were none.

Being simple in seemingly complex situations can often yield results.

Sometimes prescriptions based on skin symptoms will have unexpected benefits on other levels, and experiences of that kind can teach you about the constitutional application of small remedies.

CASE 7

A woman of 38 with eczema and dermographic skin. She is a highly strung person who often weeps during the consultation without knowing why. Over a period of six years it had been difficult to find a remedy that suited her really well constitutionally, although she had benefited from Sepia and Ignatia. She was prescribed Mezereum on the basis of the following symptoms:

> HEAD; ERUPTIONS; itching
> SKIN; ERUPTIONS; scratching, after
> SKIN; ITCHING; eruption; without
> SKIN; ITCHING; warm, becoming
> GENERALITIES; heated, becoming

This had a dramatic effect, not only on the skin, but also on her nervous state. She previously had a general jumpiness and free-floating anxiety that was difficult to relate to anything in particular. It was therefore not easily interpreted into rubrics. Mezereum is a fascinating remedy and has a profound effect on the nervous system (see the materia medica chapter, page 119).

Many useful 'eczema remedies' will be found by paying particular attention to the skin symptoms where there is a paucity of characteristic mental and general symptoms. Remedies such as Clematis, Mezereum, Oleander, Petroleum, Sarsaparilla or Viola Tricolor will be difficult or even impossible to arrive at by any other means.

SUPERFICIAL SYMPTOMS, SUPPRESSION
AND PROVING

In Paragraph 7 of the *Organon*, Hahnemann talks of 'the short-sighted method called symptomatic therapy' in which symptoms are suppressed. He says, 'A single symptom is no more the whole disease than a single foot a whole man.' He is referring here to allopathic medicine, 'The Old School' and the use of 'the opposite remedy'. It is also true of homoeopathy that it is almost always impossible to prescribe successfully on the basis of a single symptom. The intelligent use of the symptom complex representing the outer manifestations of disease in the analysis of a case can be an invaluable strategy, as has already been discussed. This is nevertheless a controversial area for homoeopaths.

Homoeopaths agree that prescribing an opposite medicine on the basis of a disease name and applying topical pharmacological treatments to skin eruptions will not be curative and will usually be suppressive. Some of them extend that concept into homoeopathic methodology, believing that the incorporation of the most superficial (skin) symptoms in the analysis will lead to the prescription of a suppressive remedy. Hopefully this chapter may help to demonstrate that skin symptoms are useful, not only as part of the totality of symptoms but because they often hold the key to resolving some very difficult situations. They are often all we have to work with – using them can lead, not to suppression, but to dramatic progess in the direction of the Law of Cure.

For all homoeopaths prescribing is an imprecise art, and at every turn one is confronted with unclear differentiations between possible remedies. Whatever method we use, we frequently give the wrong remedy. To the novice prescriber it is important to stress that even the most experienced homoeopath does that. Teaching situations often give the impression that the experts never make mistakes and this can be discouraging to beginners. It can also result in practitioners becoming disappointed in themselves when they cannot achieve consistently good results.

The administration of inappropriate remedies is as likely to occur using the methods described in this book as with any other technique. The question is, what happens when we choose the wrong remedy, particularly when it is based mostly, or totally, on skin symptoms?

It seems there are two answers to this question and a large grey area in between. The most common answer is based largely on adopted principles and belief systems:

(a) The result will either be suppression or a 'spoiled case'.

After thousands of consultations I am still looking for evidence of suppression and spoiled cases as a result of homoeopathic treatment. If you rigidly adopt any set of beliefs you are likely to interpret observations or clinical experience in a way that supports those beliefs. The whole question of beliefs and the role they play in what we do is a complex subject. It could shed light on why concepts which are very real to homoeopaths go unnoticed by allopaths (for example, Hering's

Law of Cure, or vaccinosis) and why some homoeopaths' patients suffer severe aggravations while those of others do not, and why organised provings produce more symptoms than incorrectly prescribed remedies. Generally speaking, homoeopaths are no different to anyone else in their dislike of discussing the extent to which belief structures play a part in their work.

The other answer, which mirrors the experience of the author (and is no doubt very much influenced by his beliefs!) is as follows:

(b) There are various possible outcomes determined by the relative dissimilarity of the remedy and the dosage scheme employed:

- Totally inappropriate remedies that are in no way suitable will have no effect at all, even if the patient persists with it for a long time. This is often seen in patients who have self-treated over long periods with Rhus Toxicodendron for rheumatism or Graphites for eczema, for example, before coming for help.

- A proving takes place. In order for there to be a proving there needs to be a degree of similarity and susceptibility. Over-persistence with a dissimilar remedy should obviously be guarded against. Hahnemann says in Paragraph 283 of the *Organon*, '...because these doses are so small, if through human weakness he chooses a medicine rather inappropriate to the disease, the harm done would be so insignificant that it would quickly be overcome and corrected by the life-force itself and the counter influence of a more similar remedy immediately administered...' This is certainly borne out in practice. The effect of a wrong remedy rarely lasts long if it is not over-prescribed and if it is followed by a more similar remedy. The use of low potencies makes situations like this relatively easier to manage. This is discussed in the Case Management chapter.

- We choose a similar remedy that is not the simillimum, or at least is not similar enough to evoke a curative response. Sometimes a partially similar remedy alters the symptom picture in a non-curative way. In this case we will either see a lateral shift in the symptoms with no amelioration or a short-lived improvement that cannot be repeated with the same remedy. The term 'lateral shift' means a change in the symptom picture, or a change of emphasis of symptoms, without an actual improvement either in the local or general symptoms.

Total suppression – to the extent that is often the case in allopathic medicine – is so rare in homoeopathic practice that it is difficult to say much about it.

There are cases that have been presented as homoeopathic suppression which could have been interpreted differently – for example, the natural course of the disease, or a situation arising in spite of the treatment rather than because of it.

MILD TO MODERATE ECZEMA CASES

These sorts of cases need little saying about them, as they are usually treated by the most common method – by using a combination of mental, general and particular symptoms. Here follow five (abbreviated) examples:

CASE 8

This child adored extra-strong mints. He was always eating them and yet he was only three years old. He was very fussy, especially about mess and dirt, and was always picking fluff off his father's clothes while he was being carried. His rubrics were:

MIND; FASTIDIOUS
SKIN; ERUPTIONS; dry; bleeding; scratching, after
GENERALITIES ; FOOD and drinks; pungent things; desires

Only one remedy is in all the rubrics: Arsenicum Album.

CASE 9

A 12-year-old boy is brought with eczema on the feet. He presents as a mild-mannered boy who takes school work very seriously. He never has to be told to do his homework and always does it to the best of his ability. He is neat and precise in the way he does things. His mother says he worries a lot – not about anything major, because they have a happy and secure home life – but about small everyday things, to a disproportionate degree. He is impatient, hates waiting for anything, and is very poor at making decisions, probably because he wants to get things right all the time. He is a chilly person. No strong food desires or aversions. His eczema is much itchier at night. The analysis was:

Anxiety about trifles
Conscientious about trifles

Impatience
Irresolution
Itch worse at night
Lack of vital heat

Four remedies run through these rubrics – Graphites, Thuja, Baryta Carbonica and Silicea. This is where a knowledge of materia medica is needed to help differentiate between the remedies. Even then, it is often a gamble and may require a process of elimination. In this case Graphites was the curative remedy. It was a rare and satisfying case in that the condition responded quickly and permanently and only required the one remedy. It was prescribed in the 12c potency, three times a day for five weeks.

CASE 10

A 32-year-old woman with eczema on her hands and wrists and nipples. The skin was cracked, often deep cracks like cuts. Her nipples were also cracked. She described herself as a secretive person. She found that unlike most of her friends she did not talk about her personal affairs to others, even to people she knew well. The only other thing she said about herself was that she did not take any nonsense from other people, although she put it more rudely. That was virtually all she said of herself – her secretiveness demonstrated itself well in the consultation. Once she referred to an ex-boyfriend as a 'bloody idiot', but that was the closest she came to talking about her personal life.

There was little to go on. The symptoms used were:

Abrupt
Secretive
Skin, cracks, deep, bloody

The remedy was Nitric Acid, which acted very well. Lycopodium, Natrum Muriaticum and Petroleum had previously been given with no effect.

Many eczema cases progress through several remedies – the so-called zigzag way to cure. In some cases it will be because the practitioner has failed to find the simillimum. In others, in my view, it is because there simply is not one simillimum. The one-remedy cases are relatively rare and are usually not serious cases.

CASE 11

A two-year-old girl with no characteristic skin modalities or symptoms was cured of eczema based on the following repertorisation:

MIND; FEAR; noise, from
EXTREMITIES; WALK; late learning to
SKIN; ERUPTIONS; eczema
GENERALITIES; FOOD and drinks; milk, desires

The remedy was Borax, which only needed to be repeated twice in the 30c potency over a three-month period.

CASE 12

A four-year-old girl with eczema in the bend of her arms, wrists and behind her knees. There were no modalities other than the itching being worse at night. She was a very clinging child. She had just started school and found it overwhelming. She was shy and got very nervous in large groups of people. She did stand up for herself though, and would retaliate in confrontations. She had a good appetite but was particularly fond of sweet things, more so than her brother. The case was repertorised thus:

MIND; TIMIDITY
EXTREMITIES; ERUPTION; joints; bends of
SKIN; ITCHING; night
GENERALITIES; FOOD and drinks; sweets, desires

The remedy was Petroleum, which worked quickly and effectively in the 200c potency.

DEFINITELY MAYBE

The frequent use of words like *usually, sometimes, often, could, might* may have been noticed in this chapter. That is because there are few strict rules in homoeopathy. At the core of our discipline are the principles that homoeopaths perceive to be unchangeable and natural laws, above all the Law of Similars and the Law of Cure. Perhaps we should formulate an additional law, the Law of Individuality. Roughly, it could state that each individual responds to his or her environment, and each disease process expresses itself, in a unique way.

Thus we recognise that there is a hierarchy in whatever symptom complex we are dealing with – the more characteristic the symptom, the more important it is. We also see that every remedy's individual symptoms have degrees of uniqueness. So at one end of the spectrum, every eczema patient has an eruption (not unique), but very few have eruptions that only itch in the open air (quite unique). Similarly, in some cases the vital force expresses its imbalance through dreams, fears and delusions, in others through physical symptoms and modalities. Some patients respond well to high potencies, others do not. Some cases aggravate, others do not. We can understand the basic principles that determine which scenario is most likely, but there must always be a margin for error – we must be ready to expect the unexpected, and above all remain flexible.

Even the Law of Similars, it must be remembered, is called the Law of Similars and not the Law of Exacts. There are degrees of similarity too. It is the *principle* of Similars that is the natural law we should adhere to. With the number of possible remedies available to us and the number of permutations and combinations of symptoms expressed in people, surely the chances of finding the simillimum for every case are fairly remote. It is a good policy, however, to act as if there is a simillimum for every case.

SUPPRESSION OR UNFOLDMENT?

Because of our knowledge of the injurious effects of suppression by allopathy, and the previously mentioned myths about the use of particulars in homoeopathic treatment leading to suppression, there is much fear of suppression amongst homoeopaths. While none of us would argue about the undesirability of suppression, the fear of it can cause confusion.

The example that general fretfulness and sleeplessness might become fastidiousness and sleeplessness between 2 a.m. and 4 a.m. is one that may 'push buttons' for some people. If the direction of cure is right, the new layer of symptoms should be less limiting than the ones that have improved. That is, they should impair the patient's quality of life less, and affect the vital functions and vital organs less. It would be more accurate to describe the 'symptoms of the person' that emerge during the process of cure as 'characteristics'.

Obviously, if an eruption disappears and the patient develops night terrors, anorexia and vertigo, the direction of cure is not correct. However, I have yet to see such an effect from homoeopathic treatment.

In very complex cases the unfolding process can be complicated. Stimulating the vital force with a homoeopathic remedy for the first time can be like opening Pandora's Box. In multi-miasmatic, allopathically treated patients it can require great courage on the part of the patient and the practitioner.

Here is an example of a case that may have been interpreted as being a suppression but which turned out successfully. It was a complex case but is presented as concisely as possible here:

CASE 13

This child, aged 2, had very severe eczema. At his first consultation he spent the whole time rolling on the floor screaming, such was his distress. The eruption was cracked, bleeding, suppurating and keeping him awake. He underwent treatment for two years, progressing through stages of Mercurius, Sulphur, Alumina and Arsenicum with a steady improvement. After about two years he was virtually eczema-free but suddenly developed periodic asthmatic attacks.

To any homoeopath this would set alarm bells ringing and I was no exception. However, when I assessed the course of events over the whole two years, what I saw was not only a steady improvement in the skin symptoms but a child that was thriving in every way. He was eating better, his sleep was now normal, he was mentally and emotionally well balanced and his immunity to colds and other acute complaints was good. I could see no other evidence for suppression and decided to treat the asthma as a new layer coming to the surface in order to be dealt with. It took six months of treatment with Phosphorus and Belladonna to raise his level of health another degree to the point that he is now free of any asthma symptoms. The child and his parents remain in contact and he is one of the healthiest, most well balanced children in his class at school, rarely getting acute illnesses and coping well when he does. Eczema and asthma are now only a memory for him.

SMALL PATIENTS AND THE SMALL TOTALITY

Observation is always an important aspect of attempting to understand an infant's case, and not least when treating infantile eczema. Often you will have little more than the appearance of the eczema and parent's observations to go on. In these situations, skin symptom matrices (as already discussed on pages 51–2) are invaluable. The following three cases are examples of a typical 'small totality in a small patient'.

CASE 14

This was an infant boy who presented with severe eczema all over his body. The eruption was in the form of thick yellow crusts that oozed a yellow discharge and bled from rubbing – the child rubbed his limbs together, apparently to relieve the itch. The eruption was worse from contact with water, and he was obviously more distressed when cold and happier when warm.

The analysis was as follows:

SKIN; ERUPTIONS; crusty; yellow
SKIN; ERUPTIONS; discharging, moist; yellow
SKIN; ERUPTIONS; washing; agg.
SKIN; ITCHING; air; cold; agg.
SKIN; ITCHING; bleeding; scratching, after
SKIN; ITCHING; warmth; amel.

The only remedy in all these rubrics is Dulcamara, which in the 30c potency quickly cleared the eczema.

CASE 15

A 1½-year-old old boy with eczema all over his body. The eczema came on two weeks after the MMR vaccine. The itch was much worse at night and when uncovered during the day. As soon as he was undressed he started scratching. The symptoms were exacerbated during dentition. He is an affectionate, fairly contented, though lively child:

SKIN; ITCHING; undressing; agg.
SKIN; ITCHING; warm, becoming
SLEEP; SLEEPLESSNESS; itching, from
GENERALITIES; VACCINATION; after

The remedies that come through this repertorisation are Mercurius, Psorinum and Sulphur. As the child had none of the generalities or behavioural symptoms of Mercurius or Sulphur, and because of a psoric family history, he was given Psorinum 200c twice in three months, which resulted in a disappearance of the eczema.

CASE 16

A two-year-old child with eczema behind his knees and in the bends of his elbows and under the arms. The worst time for the itching was in bed when he woke up in the morning. The eruption was not bad to look at until he started scratching, which would bring it up badly. One fingernail and two toenails had flaked off. He had a passion for milk. He was a somewhat restless child but had no marked mental or general symptoms. The rubrics chosen were:

EXTREMITIES; ERUPTION; joints; bends of
EXTREMITIES; NAILS; affections of; exfoliation
SKIN; ERUPTIONS; scratching, after
SKIN; ITCHING; morning; bed, in
GENERALITIES; FOOD and drinks; milk, desires

The remedy was Rhus Toxicodendron which, given in the 30c and later the 200c potency, resulted in a complete disappearance of the eczema.

A CAUTION: SEEK THE BIGGEST TOTALITY

Despite everything that has been said so far about the usefulness of the small totality, we should never be content with the perspective of the ant when we could have the view of an eagle. We need to beware of focusing too much on the skin and not enough on the person. This can happen as a result of lazy case-taking and a lack of insight on the practitioner's part. Some patients may also play a part in shifting the focus away from the true centre of gravity – they may not like talking about their emotions and personal life, or simply lack the self-awareness to be able to do so. It may also be that they have not been alerted to the importance of this part of the process, considering details of their physical symptoms to be more important. This is not unreasonable in the case of someone who is new to homoeopathy.

CASE 17

A 26-year-old woman with eczema on her face. The skin cracked and was worse from getting wet. The rash was very itchy, especially at night. She gave her symptoms in an abrupt manner, in the way that suggested she was irritated by the questioning. She kept saying she was perfectly healthy and normal in every other respect. She said she was easygoing and happy-go-lucky. She had not felt her normal self since giving birth two years previously.

She was given Lycopodium, Mezereum, Sepia and Tuberculinum, all with no effect. One of the things she always stressed was how much better she felt for vigorous exercise – it was one of the reasons she was given Sepia in the first place. That, together with her abrupt, almost secretive manner led to her being prescribed Ignatia, even though it is not thought of as being an 'eczema remedy'. After six weeks her skin had improved a lot. She then said: 'There is something I should have told you a long time ago. I had a termination seven years ago and I have just realised that this is at the core of my problems. I have been harbouring intense guilty feelings all this time but have never been able to bring myself to talk about it.' There was a very strong element of guilt and unresolved grief in the case which had been overlooked. Over the course of the next few months there was a coming to terms with her emotions and a simultaneous improvement of her skin.

It took the Ignatia to get this case moving. It opened it up in a way that only the simillimum could, revealing the true nature of the problem which was then able to be resolved. Her core symptoms were grief and guilt. In the consultations she succeeded, whether consciously or unconsciously, to deflect attention away from her and on to the physical problems. This case also demonstrated a weakness in the practitioner's case-taking ability.

SYMPTOMS AS SYMBOLS, ILLNESS AS METAPHOR

Taking the broader view, it is often possible to see a pattern, and thus a reason, in the symptomatology. By 'reason' we do not mean the name of the infecting organism, or which specific allergen is involved, but rather the symbolic meaning of the symptoms and how they make sense within the context of the whole – the constitution and life circumstances of the patient. This is best illustrated with a few examples.

- The patient who as a child had parents in the diplomatic service. They were never in one place for very long and his school years therefore were spent continually being uprooted and having to adjust to new circumstances. In adulthood he has been a perpetually discontented person, always frustrated by feelings of 'the grass being greener on the other side of the fence'. There is a family history of tuberculosis. This small description suggests Tuberculinum straight away. The two main characteristics of his eczema were:

Itching, changing place on scratching
Itching, wandering

It can be seen how the skin symptoms reflect the patient and in turn the indicated remedy.

- The Ignatia patient who, when asked what sort of food she likes says, 'There are swings in what I like' – a reflection of the changeability of Ignatia symptoms. Ignatia patients will often use expressions like 'up and down' when asked how they are.

- The Belladonna patient who described her eczema as 'Hitting me every summer – I fight it with hydrocortisone but the attacks are more vicious every year.' The eruption was 'angry' and bright red and inflamed. The language suggests being in a battle and the rubrics that were used in the analysis were:

  MIND; DELUSIONS; war, being at
  MIND; TALK, talking, talks; battles, about
  SKIN; ERUPTIONS; rash; scarlet
  SKIN; INFLAMMATION
  GENERALITIES; SEASONS; summer; agg.

- The Natrum Muriaticum patient who 'could not face' her employer after being reprimanded at work. She developed eczema all over her face which prevented her from attending work, as appearance was important in her particular role. The remedy cleared the skin and resolved the emotional disturbance.

- The patient with chronic catarrh and eczema that appears only on uncovered parts, who finds it impossible to access her feelings or talk about her emotions, and who as a child saw a dead body being dragged from a lake. The remedies were Staphysagria and Thuja. The theme of the case was 'that which is hidden, covered and suppressed', which are important aspects of the two remedies that helped her.

- The Sepia patient who constantly talked of life as being too pressurised. She suffered from terrible headaches with pain as if her head was in a vice, and eczema in places where tight clothing rubbed. Her husband was rather immature and she often referred to how he was like a third child to her.

This way of looking at things involves practitioner interpretation, which can be a dangerous filter through which to process information. It can lead to self-delusion so – as with every approach – it should not be forced onto every case. Reading some meaning into everything can be misleading. Just as a fake psychic will usually find someone in the audience who will verify most of their insights, we can often find ways of making symptoms fit metaphors where convenient. I remember reading something by a Buddhist Lama, who said 'Everything that happens has meaning, but try and interpret it at your peril.'

REVERSE ELIMINATION

Some remedies have such strong, reliable modalities that the absence of such a symptom can be used to eliminate a remedy that may be suggesting itself in other ways. Some examples of this are:

Where Rhus Toxicodendron suggests itself but the itch is not ameliorated by warmth.

Sulphur suggests itself but the itch is not aggravated by warmth.

Mercurius suggests itself but the itch is not worse at night.

Alumina or Petroleum seem indicated but the eruption is not worse in winter.

Some symptoms are common to eczema and their absence can lead you to remedies that are not listed in the appropriate rubric. It is relatively common for the itching of eczema to be worse at night. Most of the well known eczema remedies and polychrests are listed in that rubric. If, for example, you have a case in which the itch is very definitely not worse at night, it will help to de-emphasise the remedies in the 'itch, worse at night' rubric and emphasise remedies like Arsenicum Album, Calcarea Carbonica and Rhus Toxicodendron, which are not in that rubric but which are otherwise indicated.

Chapter 4

Reasons for Failure

EDUCATING THE PATIENT

The Time Factor – Impatient Patients

It is important to be clear from the beginning what sort of timescale you consider will be necessary in order to:

1) get enough improvement to gain the patient's confidence, and
2) effect a cure or amelioration of the presenting complaint sufficient for the patient's long-term needs.

Provided that the homoeopathic evaluation has been done well, the most common reason for failure in eczema cases is where the patient gives up the treatment prematurely. Of course this is something that can too easily be used as an excuse for failure, and we all have patients who have persevered without benefiting. However, with eczema, early frustration and consequent cessation of treatment is not unusual. It is easy to forget that many of the people who come for help have expectations moulded by their experience of allopathic treatment. Conventional dermatology has perfected many quick-acting suppressive treatments, and most eczema sufferers have only that approach as a reference. They are conditioned into expecting an overnight disappearance of symptoms. They may want the same effect from your treatment as they get from applying hydrocortisone. It is therefore important to prepare the patient so that they know, in most cases, that it is not going to be an overnight process.

It is rare, in long-standing eczema in adults, to achieve lasting and substantial improvement in less than one year. It is wise to suggest to the patient that it may take one to two years to achieve a substantial result in a chronic case, even though more recent problems can be quicker to resolve. Infants need at least six months of treatment. That is not to say that it will always take so long to get an improvement – symptoms can reduce very quickly – but to achieve a lasting cure does take time.

By being clear about this from the outset, the patient can decide whether they want to commit themselves or not. While perseverance does not guarantee success, it is often necessary in order to achieve significant improvement with a condition like eczema.

A dissatisfied patient who gives up treatment is the worst outcome for everybody. It results in the patient getting no relief from their suffering, wasting their money, forming a negative view of homoeopathy (which may be passed on to others), and leads to frustration and quite possibly a poor reputation for the practitioner. We therefore owe it to our patient, ourselves and to homoeopathy in general to have an understanding of what will be involved.

You can never be sure what would have happened if a patient who gave up treatment had persevered, but the following case is an example of one that almost certainly could have been helped more than was possible with allopathic treatment.

CASE 18

He was a very restless child of the sort that makes a consultation difficult. He would keep escaping from the room and his mother would have to chase after him. He was always moaning and complaining and very difficult to please, never satisfied for long. When angry he would strike his head against the floor or wall, and had the habit of biting other children. He had a strong desire for bananas which, although not in Kent's *Repertory* is a verified addition to *The Complete Repertory*, and is a symptom for the remedy he needed. The rubrics relevant to the case were:

MIND; BITING
MIND; DISCONTENTED; displeased, dissatisfied
MIND; RESTLESSNESS; nervousness; children, in
MIND; STRIKING; knocking his head against wall
GENERALITIES; FOOD and drinks; bananas; desires

Tuberculinum is the only remedy in all these rubrics. You would not really need to repertorise this case, so clear is the picture of that remedy.

It was explained to the child's mother that the chances of a cure were very good indeed and all that was required was patience in order for him to do well on homoeopathic treatment. There was quite a lot of potential for aggravation in the case because the child's energy was very vital and reactive and the eruption had been subject to suppression with hydrocortisone.

It was therefore decided to start him on Tuberculinum 6c, three times a day. After two weeks his mother rang to say that he was much worse, upon which she was told to cease the administration of the remedy for a few days to let things settle down. She then resumed the remedy but only gave it twice a day. Once again the eruption aggravated unexpectedly badly but calmed down again when the remedy was stopped. What surprised his mother was the extent to which the boy calmed down and became much less aggressive and restless during this period. His appetite also improved. This of course confirmed that the remedy was acting curatively and that the apparent worsening of the skin was part of the healing process.

However, the child's parents lost faith and despite reassurance did not like the way the skin was reacting to the treatment. There was little more that could have done to avoid aggravation, and the technique being used would, in most cases, not have resulted in such violent aggravation. It was something that needed to be worked through, and it probably would not have taken more than a further month of treatment to get improvement. The parents reverted back to allopathic treatment.

A few months later the boy was admitted to hospital with a severe asthma attack. He did not suffer from asthma when he first came for treatment, and it is almost certain that this was a consequence of the suppression of his eczema. It is a sad story because the child had a very good chance of having his general level of health improved by homoeopathy but instead he got the opposite – quite possibly a lifetime on asthma drugs.

Suppressing Aggravation

The question as to what extent suppression prevents or impairs the healing process is also addressed in Chapter 5. The possibility of aggravation is one of the most important things to warn the patient of. It is also one of the concepts most familiar and acceptable to people new to homoeopathy. The idea of 'getting worse before you get better' even appeals to some people. Maybe it is because of the notion that something is 'coming out', almost like an exorcism of something unpleasant from the body. Some people accept it because it is, at least, a tangible sign that indicates that these strange pills containing 'nothing' are actually doing something.

It is therefore not often that a patient will aggressively suppress an aggravation of symptoms by using hydrocortisone or other medication, but it does happen. To suppress an aggravation will antidote the effect of the remedy, at least partially and most often totally. Make sure to advise against such a course of action.

Lifestyle and Diet

Sometimes homoeopaths place too much reliance on their remedies and overlook the part that external factors play in the case.

There is the other side of the coin too. You will frequently be consulted by patients who have tried other types of therapists, including clinical ecologists, nutritionists and naturopaths. These approaches sometimes see eczema as being entirely a food allergy problem. Some eczema patients benefit from this approach but it is usually only palliative and depends on maintaining a strict dietary regime. Probably the best approach is to be aware of the possibility of food sensitivity, but to consider it as part of the syndrome of which the eczema is also part. As such it can be a maintaining cause that will impair the action of remedies and the progress of cure, but is not an end in itself.

There exists a school of thought that considers cow's milk to be the major 'cause' of eczema. Many Tubercular children will benefit from moderating their milk intake. A severe sensitivity to milk will act as a very strong obstacle to cure. If the existence of such a sensitivity is unclear, it can be worth having a trial milk-free period of, say, three weeks to see whether the skin symptoms calm down. Many children who have been put on strict dairy-free diets have not benefited, so routine dietary advice is not recommended. The other main culprit in the food line is wheat. In the most stubborn cases it is worth trying a period on a wheat-free and dairy-free diet.

Allergy tests are notoriously unreliable, although the most recent developments, like Elisa IgG testing, are refining the procedure. The most reliable method of testing is by food elimination. It is rare for there to be a wide variety of foods aggravating eczema, but it should always be borne in mind if seemingly well indicated remedies are not working as effectively as expected.

One of the most powerful maintaining causes is emotional stress. There is a variety of experience one can have regarding this:

1) Patients who either, as a result of the treatment, or by talking to their homoeopath, become aware of the part stress is playing in the situation and endeavour to do something to alleviate the situation.
2) Those who are aware that there is a stress component but either consider it to be unimportant or something that cannot be changed and just has to be put up with.

3) Sometimes the practitioner senses that there is more to the situation than meets the eye but is not able to confirm suspicions regarding, for example, family dynamics and the part that emotional stress is playing in the person's illness. This may be because the patient is deliberately concealing information, or because they are in a state of denial and are not able to access their feelings.

Emotional and mental stress may either be the exciting cause or a maintaining cause of the eczema. Either way, failing to reveal the full nature of that stress, or omitting to deal with it by some means other than homoeopathic remedies, will limit the progress of the case.

THE ELUSIVE SIMILLIMUM

The most obvious and common reason for failure, in all types of case, is the inability to find the correct remedy for the patient. However, it must be stressed that there is not always one remedy that has to be pursued like the Holy Grail. There will be cases where flexibility is required as you work through the stages of treatment. It may be necessary to use a series of remedies over a period of time. The one-remedy case does occur, but only about 50% of the time. The 'zigzag' way to cure is less satisfying in some ways but is often the only way, whether it be through the practitioner's lack of ability or the complexity of the case. It is a good approach, however, to act as if there is an elusive simillimum that has yet to be found, as this encourages conscientious case analysis. Again, it must be mentioned for the sake of beginners, that every homoeopath, even the most famous, has many 'zigzagged' cases in their files.

LOOKING FOR POLYCHRESTS

In one-sided cases, especially those of infants, it is easy to be drawn into trying to make every case fit one of the well-known polychrests. Thus placid babies are given Calcarea Carbonica, friendly affectionate ones, Phosphorus, when in fact they may need a remedy that has no mental symptoms but has characteristic skin symptoms.

CASE 19

A nine-month-old baby presented with eczema all over his body. He is a happy, cheerful child and has been very easy to look after. Good pregnancy and birth, healthy appetite, walked at eleven months etc. His symptoms were:

Itching worse at night
Pain after scratching (cries after scratching)
Moist eruption behind ears (where it first appeared – it only spread after this was suppressed)
Aversion to cheese

The remedy was Oleander – a remedy that does not normally have prominent mental symptoms. Note that Calcarea Carbonica eczema is rarely markedly worse at night.

LATERAL THINKING – NON-REPERTORIAL PRESCRIPTIONS

Some of the most intractable cases are ones in which we have relied too much on the precision of the repertory. Certain curative remedies will only be found by thinking laterally and putting a different interpretation on our repertorisations. This is particularly true of some mineral remedies. If, say, Aurum Metallicum and Sulphur both feature strongly in the case and neither has helped entirely on its own, you may need Aurum Sulphuricum. Similarly, if Lachesis features strongly but does not act curatively, be aware of smaller snake remedies that may be coming through the repertorisation. Computer expert systems can help suggest such remedies.

In most cases, if an unusual remedy is to be found by this method it will appear in one or two of the symptoms in your repertorisation, as well as being suggested in the above ways. The exceptions to this are of course unproved remedies such as Baryta Nitrica and Calcarea Muriatica, but these are not likely to be needed in more than a very small percentage of cases.

INFLEXIBILITY

It is a real skill to be able to judge with certainty when the remedy needs to be changed and when it needs to be given longer to act. This is the skill of the selection of 'the second prescription' – that is, the one after the one that has acted. From the case analysis chapter it should be clear that the fact that a particular remedy has brought about an improvement does not necessarily guarantee that it is also going to complete a cure.

Positively persisting with a remedy when it is no longer appropriate, simply because 'it worked before so it should work again', will lead to frustration and failure. Failure may also arise from changing remedies prematurely and being impatient. Similarly, adhering strictly to rules such as 'never repeat Lachesis within three months' is, in the author's experience, more limiting than helpful.

There is a delicate balance to be struck between over-prescribing and under-prescribing. It is necessary to keep up the momentum in the healing process, yet not to push too hard. Only very careful attention to detail in follow-ups will make it possible to know when to repeat the remedy, give a different one, change the potency or give nothing at all. Most classical homoeopaths have a fear of overprescribing and will tend to wait rather than risk giving a remedy prematurely. This is an important principle which should always be taken into consideration – the principle of the minimum dose. However, time can be wasted and patient confidence lost by erring too much on the side of caution.

GOING TOO DEEP

There is the scenario in which the patient feels generally better and improves in other ways but the skin stays the same or gets worse. There are different models you can apply to explain this phenomenon. The concept of layers is a useful one. If you prescribe on 'too deep a layer' it will often cause aggravation of the skin symptoms with no subsequent amelioration. This is indicative of a case where it may be necessary to 'treat the skin' – the lesion layer – before treating the person on a deeper level. It is in cases like this where small remedies are often appropriate. This idea of 'going too deep' is a mistake commonly made by Kentian and psychologically oriented practitioners. It is an error encouraged by the philosophical belief that particular symptoms and symptoms of the skin are not relevant to the case analysis, or that using them may be suppressive.

Prescribing nosodes early on in treatment on the basis of family history and miasmatic influence can cause aggravation without amelioration. Sometimes it is necessary to give the indicated remedy before nosodes are used. In other cases, where there are only indications for a nosode it is perfectly acceptable to open with one. However, in such cases there will usually be symptoms that suggest the nosode as a remedy – that is, indications more complex than just family history and miasmatic influence.

BEING TOO SHALLOW

Another scenario is where we focus too much on the skin and not enough on the person. This may be through the practitioner's lack of insight or it may be that the patient plays a part in shifting the focus away from the true centre of gravity. It cannot be stressed enough that while this book discusses the use the symptoms of the skin in case analysis, many cases will not require such an approach. Superficial prescribing is an error made by poorly trained homoeopaths and those who use specifics, or therapeutics, and prescribe on keynotes. There are homoeopaths who, without realising it, adopt an almost allopathic approach in their assessment of their patients. Whether you use potentised homoeopathic material or allopathic medicines, viewing patients and their disease in a non-holistic way will not produce deep cures.

The concept of physical symptom matrices, as mentioned in the Case Analysis chapter, can also be used incorrectly. To look no further than the symptoms of the skin in a case that is rich in mental and general symptoms will lead to failure. Indeed, if homoeopathic suppression is at all possible, this is the way it is most likely to occur. For example, a case of eczema presents as fissured and exuding a sticky honey-like fluid. These symptoms suggest Graphites; however it would not be an appropriate prescription if the patient was an angry, confrontational person with a fear of heights and who loved sweets and salt. It would more probably be Natrum Muriaticum or Sulphur in this case.

HYDROCORTISONE

Of all the drugs our patients may be on, nothing quite has the antidoting effect of steroid medication. Even as a topical application it can be a strong obstacle to cure, especially if it has been used liberally and over a long period of time. It should not however, be withdrawn suddenly, and optimally under the guidance of the patient's general practitioner. The rebound effect of doing so and prescribing remedies at the same time can cause unmanageable aggravation. See the next chapter for further advice on this subject.

In the most stubborn cases, with a history of much steroid use, it may be necessary to give hydrocortisone in potency to remove the block created by the drug. Its effect on impairing the immune system's ability to respond to homoeopathic remedies is a real problem in many cases.

INCURABLE CASES

A certain combination of factors may produce a situation in which a successful outcome is virtually impossible. Adults who have had eczema since childhood, and who have used a lot of suppressive treatment all their life, have a poor prognosis. The cumulative effect of years of steroid use can result in a powerful rebound effect once homoeopathic treatment begins. It is only the most trusting patient who would be prepared to persevere for five or more years with only slight progress, and possibly much suffering, in order to cure their eczema. Even the most careful management and great tolerance on the patient's part may not be sufficient to reach a satisfactory conclusion.

Add to many years of suppression an unfortunate combination of miasmatic influences, and the situation can become impossible. Even in children, a very complicated family history with two or more miasms strongly present can result in a perplexing case, in which significant progress without serious aggravation is very difficult – and sometimes even impossible – to achieve. There are 'anti-miasmatic' prescribing methods involving the use of many remedies in short succession that claim to be particularly useful in these complicated cases. Despite researching such claims I have seen little evidence that they are any more effective than more classical approaches.

Incurability may be an inappropriate term; maybe insufficient time, patience and tolerance is a better way of expressing it. In the worst cases we have to respect the sufferer's inability to cope with years of rebound reaction, aggravation, itching, suppuration and other complications. It is worth considering, even if difficult to accept, that for some a lifetime on hydrocortisone could give a better quality of life than attempting to cure the condition with homoeopathy with all that that entails.

Chapter 5

Aggravation and Case Management

COMMONSENSE PRECAUTIONS

There is a certain amount of simple self-care that can make a difference even before treatment begins. The patient should be encouraged to take note of the following:

- Use cotton sheets to avoid overheating and perspiration in bed.
- Wear cotton clothes and avoid wool, as well as artificial fibres.
- Wash clothes in non-biological and preferably unperfumed washing powders, and do not use fabric conditioners.
- Avoid perfumed soaps and bubble baths.
- After swimming in chlorinated water, have a shower and apply an emollient.
- If the hands are affected, use gloves for household chores, gardening, DIY, etc.
- Protect young babies from direct sun but avoid alcohol-based sun blocks.
- Keep children's fingernails cut as short as possible and use mittens if necessary.
- Vacuum clean mattresses and keep the bedroom as dust-free as possible, as dust-mite allergy is common in atopics.
- Avoid foods that appear to provoke or aggravate the condition. (See also pages 75 and 90.)

PREDICTING AGGRAVATION

The nature and likelihood of aggravation is difficult to predict. There are four main factors to consider when assessing the potential for aggravation:

1) The extent of the history of suppression in the case. There can be a rebound effect where an eruption has been aggressively suppressed. The more difficult the eruption was to suppress, the more violent the rebound is likely to be once the curative process begins. Severe

cases that have required hospital treatment in the past can be very problematic and require a lot of skill and caution on the homoeopath's part.

2) The vitality of the patient. A fiery, high-energy person is more likely to produce a strong aggravation than a slow, phlegmatic person.

3) Linked to this is the nature of the remedy being prescribed. There are remedies that are great 'unsuppressors' – remedies with a particularly strong 'centrifugal action'. For example, Belladonna, Lachesis, Psorinum, Staphysagria, Sulphur and Zincum. Remedies one would expect to have a less violent effect are Alumina, Calcarea Carbonica, Clematis, Pulsatilla and Silicea. It can be seen that some of the 'unsuppressors' are remedies that have a fiery nature – thus the link between factors (2) and (3).

4) The 'miasmatic roots' of the condition. Assessing the patient's family history is important for the sake of establishing what lies within the Pandora's box of the patient's constitution. Being aware of this, and taking into consideration the above factors, can help one to determine how slowly the box should be opened!

Even after evaluating the above factors it is prudent to be sparing in one's predictions of prognosis to patients, and to err on the side of caution. The following examples show two sides to the unpredictable nature of response to treatment.

CASE 20

A patient who had eczema on his hands for at least twenty years. He was a labourer who had spent his life working outdoors building roads. A few years previously allopathic treatment removed the eczema from his hands and it had subsequently reappeared on his face.

He presented a fairly clear picture of Sulphur and with that remedy alone his eczema cleared up in three months with no aggravation at all. This is unusual, considering the history of suppression and the length of time he had had the complaint. However, what was striking about this patient was how simple and down-to-earth he was. In Britain we do not have a 'peasant class' any more, but this man was the closest thing to being a 'peasant' that you might find. That is not meant in a derogatory sense, but more in terms of how rustic and uncomplicated he was. He was like someone from a former age, very close to the earth, and he spent his life digging it. Maybe the fact that he responded so efficiently and without complications tells us something else about the factors that determine the response to treatment.

Sometimes there are unpleasant surprises, despite one's best efforts to avoid aggravation. This is especially true when using nosodes:

CASE 21

A case of a child with eczema that had responded temporarily to Sulphur 30c without any aggravation. On the basis of the family history and the shortness of the amelioration from Sulphur, the Sulphur was followed by Psorinum 6c to be taken twice a day. After the first dose of Psorinum the child erupted as never before. The skin became infected and she was given Calendula 30c to bring the aggravation under control. There was no amelioration after the aggravation subsided, and the parents were discouraged and did not return. It was one of those frustrating experiences that happens to every practitioner at some time.

It is difficult to know for sure what would have happened if treatment had been continued. It is possible that the Sulphur would have worked more effectively after the Psorinum. It may be that the Psorinum was a close remedy but not the simillimum, or that the Psorinum 'layer' was too deep to be treated at that time (which may be another way of saying the same thing). Some might also suggest that the Sulphur had acted suppressively and the Psorinum was undoing that. Such effective suppression from a single dose of Sulphur is extremely unlikely, however. It is rare and unexpected for a single dose of a 6c potency to have such a violent effect.

Sometimes unexpected skin eruptions occur as an initial response to treatment of other conditions:

CASE 22

A man who came for treatment of asthma. He worked in a bank and was a very proper, well-mannered person. His asthma was worse in dry weather and worse between 2 a.m. and 4 a.m. The indicated remedy was Kali Carbonicum. The asthma improved very quickly, but as it did he started developing an eruption around his eyes. The eruption got worse and worse until his eyes were all swollen and red. The skin around his eyes was desquamating and emitted a sticky discharge. It was decided to wait and let the process run its course for as long as possible.

He had an important job which involved travelling around to different branches of the bank every week, dealing with bank managers he had never met before, and he found this awful eruption on his face embarrassing under the circumstances. When it became clear that the eruption was not going to subside on its own within a reasonable time, it was decided to prescribe Graphites, which quite quickly calmed it down. The flakiness of the skin took about three weeks to disappear. He did not have a return of the asthma symptoms.

Who can say why the eruption came out around his eyes? No one could possibly have predicted that, and one wonders what future problems the appearance of that eruption might have prevented.

POTENCY, DOSAGE AND AGGRAVATION

Potency

The single most useful thing to master with regard to the avoidance of aggravation is the use of low potencies. There are exceptions, as we have already seen in Case 21, but to a great extent aggravation can be avoided if you select a low potency. At the very least, the duration of any aggravation will be lessened. By using a low potency repeated daily, cases are more manageable than if you use a medium to high potency in a single dose. By stopping the remedy, or reducing the frequency of repetition, you can very quickly slow down the response to the remedy. Obviously if you give, say, a 200c in a single dose and the patient overreacts, you either have to wait and let the patient suffer or enter into the messy, complex scenario of antidoting and treating the aggravation, which will make a difficult job even more complicated.

Low potencies, for our purposes, are defined as being between 6c and 12c. Sometimes a 6x (D6) or 3c is an appropriate starting point if the potential for aggravation is very high. The recommended frequency of the scale is 6c – 12c – 30c – 200c. In cases where aggravation occurs despite starting low, intermediate potencies can be used 6c – 9c – 12c –15c – 18c, etc. If treatment is begun at the lowest end of the scale of potencies, it is quite rare with eczema to have to go as high as 200c, and very rare to go higher than that.

LM Potencies

The LM potencies are also good in terms of their manageability and gentleness. In the event of aggravation with their use, Hahnemann recommended that the remedy be reduced and repeated at longer intervals, or even suspended for several days (*Organon*, Paragraph 248). Some practitioners prefer them to the centesimal scale, considering them to be more Hahnemannian, owing to the idea of the ever slightly altered dose. They can be given between twice a day and once a week, depending on the susceptibility of the patient. A good general starting point is once a day, with the view to tailoring the dose to the patient's needs. Experience suggests that the same results can be achieved with both the centesimal and the LM potency scales and that only personal preference and ability need determine which one to use.

Those who prefer the LM potencies believe they were Hahnemann's most recent development and as such supersede the centesimal potencies. The LMs are administered in water and succussed with each administration. This satisfies the idea that the vital force 'does not accept an unchanged dose without resistance' (*Organon*, Paragraph 246). LMs are more dilute and subject to more succussion than centesimals. This combination may be why they seem to be both deep-acting and gentle at the same time. One of their other advantages, as with the low centesimals, is that they are easier to manage. Over-reaction will subside quickly on cessation of the remedy.

Some practitioners are put off by the seemingly complicated means of administration of the LMs. The traditional method is to dissolve one granule in about 150 ml of water and alcohol. The patient succusses this each time and adds one teaspoon to a glass of water. The glass of water is then stirred vigorously and a teaspoon dose taken from it. Most people who have significant experience of using them find that it is acceptable to take a few drops directly from the stock bottle rather than dilute it each time. This makes their use more convenient and means that the patient can carry a small dropper bottle with them for use during the day if necessary.

It appears to be best to begin with LM1. In most cases, increasing the potency by one degree every four weeks works well. However, the needs of the individual always determine the dosage scheme. Some may be able to stay on the same potency for two months or more, whereas others will need to increase it after three weeks.

Repetition of the Dose

How much remedy to give is a constant topic of debate amongst homoeopaths.

Hahnemann states in the *Organon* and *Chronic Diseases* his belief that the dose should not be repeated while the preceding one is acting:

> 'Every perceptibly progressive and strikingly increasing amelioration during treatment is a condition which, as long as it lasts, completely precludes every repetition of the administration of any medicine whatsoever ...' *Organon*, Paragraph 246.

'... it is important to observe, that our vital principle cannot well bear that the same unchanged dose of medicine be given even twice in succession, much less more frequently to a patient.' (*The Chronic Diseases*)

The experience of the Argentinian homoeopath Francisco Eizayaga contradicts this view. This can be studied in detail in his *Treatise on Homoeopathic Medicine*. It is similarly my experience that low potencies can be repeated frequently and continued while amelioration is under way. No explanation can be offered as to why Hahnemann felt 'plussing' was essential if the dose was to be repeated frequently. Many homoeopaths have now successfully adopted the use of repeated doses of the centesimal potencies and have verified the efficacy of the repetition of the unchanged dose for as long as it is appropriate.

In most eczema cases the potency will only need to be increased every six to twelve weeks. If the interval is nearer six weeks, then the potency was probably a little lower than optimum. If the potency continues to act for ten, twelve or more weeks, it is the simillimum of potencies.

It is recommended that the remedy, if in the 6c or 12c potency, be given between two and three times a day. It appears that if the remedy is the simillimum, the vital force will take as much as it needs to begin the curative process and that all subsequent doses will act as placebo. As the effect of the previous dose wears off, the vitality will automatically begin to use the subsequent doses being regularly administered. It is sometimes asked why patients taking repeated doses do not prove the remedy. The reason appears to be that a proving will not take place while the remedy being taken is still indicated.

There is much that we do not understand about the action of dynamised medicines. It is surely wiser to base our practice on experience rather than beliefs.

Too Deep a Layer

Using either the model of layers or degrees of pathology, as already described by the plant analogy, it is possible to cause aggravation by prescribing a remedy out of sequence. Another way of describing this is in terms of Eizayaga's concept of 'constitutional, fundamental and lesional' layers. Those layers need to be treated in reverse order. To do otherwise can have the effect of 'stirring things up' without permitting a resolution.

Getting this right every time is an unrealistic expectation to have of oneself. Layers and the plant analogy are easier to understand when described as concepts. However, differentiating between layers and perceiving clearly what is uppermost in the case can be difficult in practice. It is hoped that the suggestions offered in the Case Analysis chapter may serve to simplify this process.

The most common mistake made along these lines is by prescribing nosodes on the basis of a miasmatic analysis of the case, and not paying enough attention to the strange rare and peculiar symptoms. By prescribing a nosode out of turn you may be bypassing between one and three other layers, and this can have the effect of causing severe aggravation without subsequent amelioration.

Waiting

Most practitioners will have had or heard of the experience of a patient taking one dose of a remedy which catalyses a reaction that continues for many months. If it is your preference to use medium to high potencies it is possible to treat eczema in this way. A case was presented at a conference in which a psoriasis patient was given a single dose of Hyoscyamus 1M. The subsequent aggravation and slow amelioration lasted for nearly two years. The only objections to this approach are that it requires tremendous patience and faith on the part of the patient and practitioner, and can sometimes cause undue suffering. Managing such situations are one of the biggest problems for relatively inexperienced practitioners.

Treating Aggravation

This is another source of confusion. In the event of an aggravation of symptoms, the ideal is to wait for it to run its course. It is advisable to strive to practise with minimum intervention. The simpler things are kept, the easier it will be to manage cases in the longer term. However, the suffering of the patient is a priority too. Remember the use of the word 'gentle' in Paragraph 2 of the *Organon*.

A very severe aggravation can run out of control. Just as a fever, while being part of a healing process, can require treatment if it goes too high, so an aggravation sometimes needs to be brought under control. There are two possibilities to be aware of:

1) If the aggravation is an intensification of the original symptoms with no significant new symptoms, then the same remedy can be given in a lower potency. The effect of this will usually be to take the intensity out of the aggravation.

2) If the symptoms of the aggravation are significantly different to the original ones, a new remedy should be selected on the basis of the new symptoms. The remedy to be used in such a situation will usually only be needed for the duration of the aggravation, but sometimes the symptoms of the aggravation will lead one to the curative remedy for the case.

Some homoeopaths advocate utilising the so-called antidoting property of coffee in such situations, but it is the author's opinion that coffee will not have any effect on a remedy which has had a significant impact on the vital force.

DETERIORATING CASES

Eczema cases rarely present problems that need conventional medical intervention. The most serious complication is infected eczema which becomes septic, and even here the correctly selected remedy will rectify the position. However, if the curative remedy is not found at once, the patient must be referred without delay for conventional treatment.

TOPICAL APPLICATIONS

Patients will often ask what they can put on their skin while they are taking remedies. It is important to tell them that all the unpleasant symptoms can be removed with internal treatment and that we do not rely on external treatments of any kind to cure the eczema. Every patient should be made aware of our views on suppression and the fact that aggressive suppression can impair or even neutralise the effect of the remedies. However, in the early stages of treatment there are things that can be done to ease the symptoms without spoiling the treatment. It is unrealistic and counterproductive to expect, for example, the patient to endure being kept awake all night with itching simply to uphold a principle. This need to make the patient 'suffer on the altar of homoeopathy' is unnecessary and unhealthy.

There are two ways in which patients will want to help themselves with topical applications:

1) The moisturising of excessively dry skin.
2) Relieving the itching

Different individuals respond to different substances. It is largely a case of finding something that suits the individual and their particular skin type. Moisturisation is a useful palliative, especially for severe itching, in the early stages of treatment, and experience indicates that it is non-suppressive.

Herbal Preparations for Topical Application

Using these is something of a hit-or-miss affair. They can be very effective for some and hardly at all for others.

Urtica Urens ointment can in some cases give relief to itchy eczema.

Calendula ointment can help in broken and infected skin. It speeds up the healing process where there is rawness and inflammation. Some people find the combination of its soothing property and the moisturising effect of the oily base of the ointment helpful.

Chickweed (*Stellaria media*) sometimes helps itching a lot. It is unreliable, though, and in severe cases seems to do little to help.

Yellow Dock (*Rumex crispus*) can similarly be excellent for palliating the itch in some cases.

There is little to differentiate between these plants, so their use is a case of trial and error.

Bach Rescue Cream sometimes has a soothing effect on itchy and painful skin.

Aloe Vera juice or gel, from *Aloe barbadensis*, which is a different species to the *Aloe socotrina* we use in homoeopathy, has been proved to have a powerful anti-inflammatory effect. It promotes skin healing and is well known for its effectiveness in speeding up the healing of burns. It can be a useful palliative in infected and raw eczema, and taken internally the juice is thought to detoxify and boost the immune system. The juice and gel are available from health food shops and chemists.

Allopathic Topical Treatments

The various allopathic treatments available for eczema have been mentioned in the first chapter of this book. By the time an eczema sufferer comes for homoeopathic treatment they have usually had experience of allopathic treatment, and will probably have found something that 'suits' their skin.

Sometimes a little suppression is not such a bad thing. Provided that internal homoeopathic treatment is also being administered, the vital force can cope with some minimal suppression from the outside. We also have to consider whether natural creams and ointments are merely inefficient suppressors. Allopathic medicine is much more adept at suppressing itch than any form of natural healing, so perhaps there is a case for using that expertise to get patients through the most difficult periods of treatment. It should, however, only be permitted where absolutely necessary – for example, where the itch is keeping the person awake or a child is scratching herself raw. Even then, ask the patient to use the absolute minimum required to make life bearable, and no more than that. Its use should be tailed off as the remedies begin to take effect. It will not be necessary for long if the internal treatment is good.

Of course, the major problem with this approach is the masking of symptoms that may be useful in the analysis of the case. Subtle modalities and sensations are easily overwhelmed by the effects of corticosteroids, so the balancing act between just enough and too much suppression is a delicate one.

DIETARY MEASURES

Apart from the possibility of food sensitivities, as discussed on page 75 under 'Lifestyle and Diet', there are other ways in which attention to diet can be helpful.

Skin irritation can be exacerbated by an acidic condition of the blood, which can be the result of eating too many acid-forming foods. The acid-alkaline balance in the body can be upset by eating a badly balanced diet. Every food is either acid-forming or alkali-forming. The average diet is acid-forming because of the quantities of sugar, coffee, dairy produce, meat and white flour that we consume.

Fruit and vegetables are alkali-forming foods. Even seemingly acidic fruits become alkaline once consumed. Fruit and vegetables have the ability to neutralise acid and detoxify the system. For this reason, even in the absence of allergies, the age-old advice of eating less junk food and more fresh fruit and vegetables can have a tangible effect in eczema sufferers. Also, homoeopathic treatment will act more efficiently in a non-toxic environment.

Organically grown and unrefined food should be encouraged as much as possible. This is likely to improve general health and reduce the toxic load on the system.

NUTRITIONAL SUPPLEMENTS

Many homoeopaths consider the use of anything other than dynamised medicines as being allopathic. Anything that raises the general level of health and increases vitality will enable the vital force and the immune system to function more efficiently. Taking appropriate nutritional supplements need be no more allopathic than eating nutritionally sound food.

Omega-6 fatty acids, the most active of which is gamma linoleic acid, and omega-3 fatty acids, which come mainly from fish, have been shown in studies to help reduce eczematous eruptions (*British Journal of Dermatology*, Nos. 113 and 117). Dry skin sufferers usually have severe omega-3 deficiency. The most effective source of both of these fatty acids in the perfect ratio is flax seed oil.

Vitamin A or beta-carotene, its precursor, are both useful in promoting cell growth and are known to improve the health of the skin. Keratin, the protein responsible for the texture and softness of the skin, needs vitamin A.

Eczema sufferers have been shown to have low levels of folic acid. It is important that they have plenty of green leafy vegetables in their diet, otherwise a supplement should be taken.

Lactobacillus acidophilus can help correct the ecology of the gut and prevent a build-up of toxins which can contribute to the severity of eczema.

The amino acids histidine and glutathione in combination have been shown to lessen the intensity of allergic eczema. Zinc supplementation up to 40mg per day has been shown to help people suffering with skin problems, including eczema and psoriasis.

None of these supplements will replace good homoeopathic treatment, but in appropriate situations they can assist the action of remedies in the same way as a clean, healthy diet.

Chapter 6

Materia Medica

This materia medica is written with the aim of facilitating the application of the remedies in eczema cases. It is what might be called an 'upside down materia medica', in that it begins with the characteristic skin symptoms and ends with the mental and general symptoms. In theory any remedy can cure skin symptoms, but it will be relatively rare to require one that is not included here in an eczema case. There are two ways in which this chapter can be of assistance.

So much has been written about the essences of the polychrests that there is little more that can be added. However, each of them have characteristic skin symptoms and 'symptom matrices' which are not described thoroughly in many other books. What is presented here is based on a combination of experience, repertory study and what has been previously written, in that order. It is the policy here to omit speculation and only include what is considered to be substantial fact. Many materia medicas, including some of the the classics, are partial reworkings of other writings and there is always something reassuring about one that is based, in the most part, on an author's personal experience.

A summary of the most important general keynotes of each remedy is also included. These symptoms are also based on the three above types of information in the same order. Conciseness of information is intentional for the sake of ease of use and comprehension. It is hoped that users will also find this a useful keynotes materia medica for all types of cases.

Secondly, there are many smaller remedies that are easily over-looked. They sometimes share combinations of symptoms with poly-chrests which makes their selection difficult, and they are invaluable if we are to be consistently effective in treating eczema. For reasons stated earlier, the idea of 'eczema remedies' is largely a taboo concept. The fact is that many small remedies have a very strong affinity for the skin and are particularly useful in severe cases. They are presented here in such a way as to make them clearly recognisable.

Careful and detailed repertorisation can make the need to memorise vast amounts of materia medica unnecessary. For example, consider the following rubrics:

SKIN; BURNING; scratching, after
SKIN; ERUPTIONS; crusty; yellow
SKIN; ERUPTIONS; discharging, moist; scratching, after
SKIN; ERUPTIONS; fissured
SKIN; ERUPTIONS; patches

These five symptoms only have four remedies in all of them: Calcarea Carbonica, Graphites, Petroleum and Viola Tricolor. The chances of arriving at Viola Tricolor without this type of repertorisation are very small.

ALUMINA

The key word is *dryness*. There is, however, a lot more to it than that, and the idea of dryness should not be allowed to eliminate it from consideration in certain other situations.

Alumina is a great polychrest with a rich picture. Its essence and mental symptoms should be understood well. It is also often possible to recognise it when there is little or no symptomatology on a mental level. This is most often the case in infants, although they will usually display some general symptom of the remedy too.

Characteristic Skin Symptoms

Dryness and roughness and thickening. Inability to perspire.
· Cracks and fissures.
Cracks that can be deep and bloody, worse for washing, worse in winter.
Eruptions worse in winter.
Dry eruptions that bleed after scratching.
Dry eruptions that discharge after scratching.
White scaly eruptions.

The Itch

Itching without eruption.
Itching worse for warmth and warmth of bed.
Itching burning after scratching. Burning alternates with itching.

93

Must scratch until it bleeds or until it is raw.
Scratching can ameliorate, aggravate, change place on scratching, or be unchanged by scratching.

Characteristic Mental Symptoms

Vague, reserved and unobserving.
Confusion as to her identity.
Difficult comprehension.
Fear of knives and blood.
Fear of insanity.
Internal hurried feeling but slowness of execution.

Most Useful General Symptoms

Chilly but worse for warmth.
Better damp, worse dryness.
Worse and averse potatoes.
Desires indigestible things, charcoal, chalk, etc.
Worse in the morning, better in the evening.

APIS MELLIFICA

Apis is well known for such conditions as erysipelas and urticaria, but is not one of the remedies first thought of for eczema. It can however be very useful in the treatment of eczema where the symptoms agree. It is important to know the chronic Apis disposition, but it also has some characteristic skin symptoms.

Characteristic Eczema Symptoms

Eruptions on perspiring parts.
Eruptions worse from cold air, even though generally worse for heat.
Red stinging eruptions.
Dermographic skin.
Dryness, desquamation and inelasticity.
Itching and stinging vesicles.
Suppressed eruptions.
Shiny red eruptions.
Swelling of affected parts.
Waxy appearance of skin.
Allergic eruptions.

The Itch

Itching worse from cold air, although generally averse to heat.
Itching on perspiring parts.
Burning and smarting.
Itch is worse becoming warm in bed.
Itching can be better for warmth (surprising in such a hot person).
The itch is usually aggravated by scratching.

Characteristic Mental Symptoms

Busy, industrious people, better when occupied.
Fruitlessly busy.
Jealousy.
Awkward, clumsy, fidgety.
Says he is well when sick.
Ailments from suppressed sexuality or sexual excess.
Ailments from anger, bad news, grief.

Most Useful General Symptoms

Aggravation from warmth of any kind - warm rooms, heat of a fire,
saunas, warm bath are all intolerable.
Right-sidedness.
Effects of suppression of any kind.
Worse from touch and pressure.
Oedematous swellings.
Thirstlessness.

ARSENICUM ALBUM

This remedy is easily recognisable because of its well-known mental
and general symptoms. It also has some very useful keynote symptoms
related to the skin that will help one to prescribe it with confidence. In
a case of severe eczema, where some of the mental symptoms like
'fastidiousness' may not be present, there is usually a general anxiety
and restlessness.

Characteristic Skin Symptoms

As many different skin symptoms as Sulphur.
Can be any of the following:
Dry and very scaly. Dry, bleeding after scratching.

Hard and thickened. Inelasticity.
Vesicular, including black and bloody vesicles.
Crusty, white or black.
Discharging, especially a corrosive discharge.
Ulcerated, suppurating.
Eruptions alternating with internal/respiratory symptoms.
Eruptions from cold air and becoming cold.
Eruptions after scratching, and thickening after scratching.
Burning after scratching.
Swelling of affected area, swelling after scratching.

The Itch

Itch better for warmth. Even scalding water ameliorates.
Itching alternating with burning.
Better when bleeding.
Worse at night.
Must scratch until it bleeds or until it is raw.
Itch usually worse scratching, can be better for scratching.
Undressing aggravates.
Itch without eruption.
Formication. Sensation of worms under the skin.

Characteristic Mental Symptoms

Insecurity, dependence.
Fearfulness – death, poverty, disease, being alone, robbers, cancer.
Fastidious, orderly and conscientious.
Censorious.
Miserly, possessive.
Restless anguish.

Most Useful General Symptoms

Restlessness.
Cold. Better warmth.
Acridity, burning sensations and discharges.
Night time aggravation, especially midnight to 3 a.m.
Periodicity.
Desires fat, sour things, cold drinks in frequent sips.
Averse to sweets (may desire), fat, farinaceous foods.
Worse for cold food, fruit, fat.

BELLADONNA

Belladonna is too often thought of as either an acute remedy or a remedy for feverish conditions. It is of course a lot more than that. It is not frequently required in the treatment of eczema, although in some severe cases can be invaluable. It is almost always indicated in plethoric individuals with a fiery nature. Children are often aggressive and fearless.

Characteristic Eczema Symptoms

Fiery red eruptions. Blotches.
Shiny eruptions like Apis.
Red streaks after scratching.
Dry burning eruptions with desquamation.
Eruptions moist after scratching.
Suppressed eruptions.
Swelling of affected parts.
Inflamed painful vesicles and vesicles that appear after scratching.

The Itch

Itching with stinging.
Itch better for scratching.
Itch unchanged by scratching.

Characteristic Mental Symptoms

Energetic, plethoric, intense temperament.
Aggressive.
Desire to bite, kick, strike, pull hair.
Strikes head against the wall with anger.
'An angel when well, a devil when sick.'
Fear of animals, dogs.
Fearlessness, audacity.

Most Useful General Symptoms

Sudden violent onset.
Right-sided.
3 p.m. aggravation.
Worse from heat, especially of the sun.
Sensitive to light, jar, noise.
Worse from suppressed perspiration, touch, motion, draughts, washing hair.

BERBERIS VULGARIS

This remedy is well known for its affinity for the urinary tract. When it is indicated in eczema cases there may be concomitant kidney symptoms. The skin symptoms can be related to a toxic or acidic condition of the system due to poor kidney function.

Characteristic Eczema Symptoms

Eruption leaves circumscribed pigmentation or brown patches.
Eruptions in patches and blotches.
Eczema on hands.
Painful red pustules.

The Itch

Itch better for cold air, water or applications.
Itch worse at night.
Itch with burning.
Scratching aggravates.
Wandering itching.

Characteristic Mental Symptoms

No mental symptoms higher than grade one in the repertory.
Darkness aggravates.
Sees forms in the dark.
Mentally exhausted.

Most Useful General Symptoms

Radiating pains.
Bubbling sensations.
Numbness.
Left-sided.
Affinity for the kidneys.

BOVISTA

The puffball is an easily overlooked remedy, but with careful repertorisation it is surprising how often it is indicated in eczema cases.

Characteristic Eczema Symptoms

Cracks and burning eruptions.
Eczema of the hands and hollow of the knees.
Eruptions bleeding after scratching.
Eruptions after scratching.
Eruptions either dry or moist after scratching.
Oozing scabs.
Burning vesicles.
Puffiness of affected parts.
Unhealthy skin, every scratch festers.

The Itch

Worse from warmth and warmth of bed.
Worse at night.
Bleeding after scratching, must scratch until it bleeds or until it is raw.
Itching with burning.
Undressing aggravates.
Itch either better, worse or unchanged by scratching.

Characteristic Mental Symptoms

Awkward in speech and action. Stammering, drops things.
Confusion.
Sensations of enlargement of parts of body.
Loquacity – open-hearted.

Most Useful General Symptoms

Tendency to puffiness.
Worse during menses.
Worse at full moon.
Worse becoming heated.
Better for eating.

CALCAREA CARBONICA

Being the major polychrest for infants and such an important anti-psoric, it is not surprising that Calcarea Carbonica is so often required for eczema. It is of course not only used for infantile eczema. In adult cases it is most often used as a 'constitutional remedy', and mostly in mild to moderate cases of eczema. It is one of the most commonly indicated remedies for eczema with itching that is not worse at night.

Characteristic Eczema Symptoms

Eruptions on the occiput, scalp and flexures.
Crusts and scabs with bland pus.
Eruptions worse from washing.
Worse in winter.
Cracking that is worse in winter.
Bleeding after scratching.
Eruptions may be: in patches, vesicular, crusty, dry and desquamating.
Milk crust.
Eruption in and around umbilicus.

The Itch

Not usually intense itching.
Itch worse in the morning in bed.
Itch on perspiring parts. Must scratch until it is raw.
Itch can be better, worse or changing place on scratching.
Worse after bathing.

Characteristic Mental Symptoms

Many fears and anxieties. Dogs, dark, death, disease, heights, poverty, insanity, animals, insects, spiders.
Obstinate.
Slowness.
Responsibility.
Sensitive hearing about cruelty.
Horrible stories affect her profoundly.
Fear of her condition being observed.

Most Useful General Symptoms

Chilly.
Worse for cold damp, change of weather.

Worse on ascending, exertion.
Worse during difficult dentition.
Sour perspiration.
Flabbiness.
Aversion to meat, milk, slimy foods, fat, coffee.
Desire for eggs, indigestible things, chalk, ice cream, starchy foods, oysters, sweets, salt, sour.
Worse from dry foods, milk.

Note: Calcarea Carbonica is in the rubric: 'Eruptions; bleeding after scratching' but not in the rubric 'Itching; must scratch until it bleeds'. The modality of the itching should not be confused with the symptom that is a characteristic of the type of eruption.

CALCAREA SULPHURICA

Calcarea Sulphurica is often thought of as a combination of Calcarea Carbonica and Sulphur. It is sometimes needed in cases that have elements of those two great polychrests, although the symptom picture should also contain unique Calcarea Sulphurica symptoms for the remedy to be indicated.

Characteristic Eczema Symptoms

Crusty eruptions, especially yellow crusts.
Unhealthy skin, poor healing, suppuration.
Pussy spots.
Dryness and desquamation – yellow scales.
Cracks.
Cracks that are worse after washing and worse in winter.

The Itch

Scratching ameliorates.
Itching with burning.
Worse on becoming warm in bed.

Characteristic Mental Symptoms

Fear of birds, the dark.
Jealousy.
Forsaken feeling.
'Lamenting because he is not appreciated.'

Most Useful General Symptoms

Tendency to suppuration.
Warm-blooded but heat, cold and damp aggravate.
Desire for open air but draughts aggravate.
Desire for green fruit.
Abscesses.
Fistulae.
Tendency to croup in children.

CARCINOSIN

Carcinosin is almost always prescribed on the basis of mental and general symptoms and the personal and familial medical history. Its effectiveness in certain cases of eczema has been confirmed in practice many times over, but few characteristic skin symptoms have emerged. It is one of the remedies for itching without eruption, and the eczema is often better by the seaside.

There are two types of Carcinosin personality, the suppressed Staphysagria sort – the sweet natured, gentle person – and there is the more extrovert, bright, energetic sort that likes dancing and being active. Both types have conscientiousness and sensitivity. The sensitivity is exhibited in the form of a sympathetic nature and sensitivity to reprimands.

Carcinosin is in the rubrics 'Ailments from admonition' and 'Offended easily' and these are common characteristics of Carcinosin children, as is also obstinacy. Fear of thunderstorms and fear of the dark may make it look like Phosphorus. The conscientiousness may also be expressed as perfectionism and an ambitious nature. Numerous strong food desires and aversions may also lead you to Carcinosin.

Do not be put off if you strongly suspect Carcinosin but there is no obvious history of it in the family – it has to start somewhere!

Characteristic Mental Symptoms

Conscientious, fastidious, perfectionistic, duty-bound.
Industrious.
Sympathetic.
Sensitive to sensual impressions.
Sentimental and affectionate.
Obstinate children.

102

Anticipatory anxiety.
Liking for animals.
Love dancing.
Love thunderstorms.
Desire for travel.
History of emotional suppression and domination.
Nail biting.

Most Useful General Symptoms

Never well since glandular fever.
Family history of cancer, TB, diabetes.
Personal history of excessive or total absence of acute disease.
Worse or better by the seaside.
Sleeps in genupectoral position or on abdomen.
Blue sclera.
Cafe-au-lait complexion.
Desires fat, eggs, chocolate, spicy, butter, fruit, salt, sweets, ice cream, vinegar.
Averse to fat, eggs, sweets, fruit, milk.

CICUTA VIROSA

Those who are not familiar with the repertory may not be aware that Cicuta is listed in black type in the rubric 'Eczema'. Cicuta has an interesting combination of mental and general symptoms, some of which will almost certainly be present in an eczema case requiring it. Childish behaviour is particularly marked in the emotional sphere.

Characteristic Eczema Symptoms

Crusty, scabby eruptions.
Crusts that form after scratching. Especially yellow crusts.
Moist eruption, discharging after scratching. Eczema madidans.
Suppuration.
Also vesicles. Confluent vesicles and pustules.
Hard thickening of the skin.
Affinity for the scalp and face.
Eczema of the scalp and meningitis.

The Itch

Often not very itchy. Can have eruption without itching.
Itching with burning.
Scratching ameliorates.

Characteristic Mental Symptoms

Childish, simple behaviour.
Suspicious.
Fear of men.
Hatred. Contempt.
Violent.
Sympathetic.
Aversion to company.
'Horrible things and sad stories affect her profoundly.'

Most Useful General Symptoms.

Tendency to convulsions, jerking and twitching.
Ailments after head injury.
Worse from touch.
Desire for chalk, charcoal, coal, indigestible things, raw potato, cabbage, alcohol.
Worse from milk.
Chilly.

CLEMATIS ERECTA

A sycotic and syphilitic remedy invaluable in any practice where skin disease often presents. It can look like one of the polychrests, especially Sulphur, as it shares some of the Sulphur modalities. It can be used in severe eczema cases where the main indications are the skin symptoms, but may also fit the case in a broader way as it has a wide spectrum of symptoms covering the urinary tract, glands, mucous membranes and eyes.

Characteristic Eczema Symptoms

Washing aggravates, especially in cold water.
Like Sulphur, can have many types of eruption:
Vesicles, itching or painful, watery or yellow.
Dry burning eruption with desquamation.
Moist and crusty with corrosive discharge.

Pustules and suppuration.
Eruptions on the occiput and lower limbs.

The Itch

Worse at night.
Worse from warmth and warmth of the bed.
Worse from cold water.
Unchanged by scratching or ameliorated by scratching.

Characteristic Mental Symptoms

Few useful mental symptoms.
Sensitive to all external impressions.
Homesickness and ailments from homesickness.
Aversion to company yet dreads being alone.

Most Useful General Symptoms

Affinity for the glands, especially testes.
Right-sided.
Effects of suppressed gonorrhoea.
Better for perspiring.

CROTON TIGLIUM

This small remedy made from croton oil seed has as its main affinities
the skin and the mucous membranes, especially of the bowel. It is one
of the remedies for complaints that alternate – for example, diarrhoea
and eruptions, or asthma and eruptions.

Characteristic Eczema Symptoms

Vesicular and pustular eruptions.
Clustered vesicles that crust when they burst.
Inflamed and scabby pustules.
Affinity for the genital region, face and head.
Alternation of eczema and internal affections.
'Sensation as if hidebound.'

The Itch

Very intense itching.
Burning and stinging.

Itching alternates with burning.
Scratching aggravates but rubbing lightly ameliorates.
Scratching in some cases ameliorates – usually light scratching.
Itch worse at night.
Warmth sometimes ameliorates.

Characteristic Mental Symptoms

Not many symptoms.
Anxiety and fear – usually associated with diarrhoea.
Selfishness, egotism.
Irritability or anxiety with the itching.

Most Useful General Symptoms

Diarrhoea that is worse from the least food or drink.
Worse for washing.
Worse in the summer.
Worse at night.
Mentally better in the open air.

DULCAMARA

Dulcamara is one of those remedies that could be called a 'minor polychrest' in that it is not used as often as, say, Lycopodium or Pulsatilla, yet has a picture that is broad and deep. Its prescription may be mainly on the basis of the characteristic skin symptoms, for example in infants, or may be based on its interesting mental and general symptoms.

Although it is not so much associated with eczema, Dulcamara's tendency to urticarial eruptions as well as to herpes must be mentioned.

Characteristic Eczema Symptoms

Crusty eruptions – moist, brown, yellow, thick.
Also pimples, pustules and vesicles.
Eruptions alternating with diarrhoea or asthma.
Washing aggravates.
Becoming cold aggravates.
Worse before and during menses.
Worse in winter.
Eczema madidans.

Eruptions that appear after scratching.
Eruptions bleed or discharge after scratching.
Skin can become hard, thick and inelastic.
Suppressed eruptions.

The Itch

Unchanged by scratching.
Worse at night.
Worse from warmth of the bed but can be better for warmth.
Worse in cold air.
Must scratch until it is raw.
Undressing aggravates.
Worse around the menses.

Characteristic Mental Symptoms

Bossy, quarrelsome.
Anxiety for others. Over-concerned about her family.
The 'mother hen'.
Scolding without being angry.

Most Useful General Symptoms

Worse for being chilled while hot.
Worse for change of temperature.
Worse for cold damp.
Worse for cold air.
Worse for suppressed discharges.
Worse in the autumn.
Better for warmth and dry weather.
Aversion to coffee.
Worse from cold food and drink.

GRAPHITES

No competent homoeopath will lack a reasonable knowledge of Graphites as a 'skin remedy', as it has been one of our greatest anti-psorics since Hahnemann's time. So characteristic are its skin symptoms that it is one remedy which can often be successfully prescribed without the use of the repertory. It is also one of the most commonly inappropriately prescribed remedies in eczema cases.

Characteristic Eczema Symptoms

Numerous symptoms but most characteristic is the honey-like, glutinous discharge.

Cracks and fissures, deep and bloody and worse in winter.

Dryness, roughness, chapping.

Moist, crusty eruptions. Crusts after scratching.

Discharge is either corrosive or fetid, offensive.

Eruptions in patches.

Itching, burning vesicles.

Eruptions alternating with internal affections.

Suppressed eruptions.

Worse before and during menses.

The Itch

Burning and prickling with itching.

Must scratch until it is raw.

Worse at night, warmth of bed.

Worse before and during menses.

Itch without eruption.

Wandering itch.

Scratching aggravates.

Characteristic Mental Symptoms

Indecisive. Timid, lacking confidence.

Fastidious, conscientious about trifles.

Fidgety.

Anticipatory.

Changeable moods.

Weeps from music.

Dullness and anxiety on waking.

Most Useful General Symptoms

Chilly, sensitive to draughts, but prone to flushes of heat.

Better open air.

Worse on waking.

Obesity.

Aggravation from suppressions.

Tendency to fissures.

Worse from bright light.

Averse to fish, salt, sweets, meat.

Desires chicken, beer.

HEPAR SULPHURIS CALCAREUM

Experience suggests that this remedy is most useful in acute stages of eczema. That is probably true of most Hepar Sulph. situations – they are usually acute or semi-acute, although the constitutional Hepar Sulph. type also exists.

Characteristic Eczema Symptoms

Cracks and painful, sensitive eruptions.
Worse in winter.
Unhealthy skin, inflammation, suppuration.
Can be dry, moist, pimples, pustules, scabs, vesicles or patches.
Fetid eruptions, especially in folds.
Thin acrid discharge.
Eruptions after scratching.

The Itch

With sticking, splinter pains.
Cold air aggravates.
Warmth ameliorates.
Must scratch until raw.
Wool aggravates.
Undressing aggravates.
Scratching ameliorates.

Characteristic Mental Symptoms

Hypersensitive and vulnerable to everything.
Irritable, impatient, hurried.
Impolite, unpleasant nature. Threatening.
Violent anger. Impulse to stab or kill.
Wants to set things on fire. Dreams of fire.

Most Useful General Symptoms

Very cold. Draught aggravates.
Uncovering aggravates.
Sensitive to pain.
Offensiveness.
Splinter-like pains.
Glandular swelling.
Worse in dry air, better for damp.

Better from warmth.
Worse in winter.
Desires vinegar, sour, spices, pungent tastes, fat.
Averse to cheese, fats.

IGNATIA

Ignatia is sometimes mistakenly thought of as only an acute grief remedy. While the root of the Ignatia state may always be in the emotions, it will not always present as an acute or a purely emotional problem. Ignatia covers virtually every imaginable disease process, not least skin symptoms.

Characteristic Eczema Symptoms

Must be mentioned for its application in urticaria from emotional causes.
Emotional aetiology.
Dryness and cracking.
Eczema around the eyes or mouth.
Blotches or vesicles.

The Itch

With stinging, burning and sticking pains.
Itch ceases with pain.
Worse from warmth.
Changes place on scratching.
Scratching ameliorates.

Characteristic Mental Symptoms

Ailments from disappointed love, disappointment, grief, anger.
Silent grief.
Suppressed anger, anger with silent grief.
Indignation, sensitive to injustice.
Idealistic, romantic.
Conscientious.
Consolation aggravates.
Alternating and contradictory states.
Easily offended, defensive.
Fear of birds.
Sighing.

Most Useful General Symptoms

Worse or better from coffee.
Worse from tobacco smoke.
Worse from cold air.
Paradoxical symptoms.
Worse from sweets.
Better from change of position and travelling.
Desires sour, bread, butter, cheese.
Averse to fruit, meat, tobacco.

JUGLANS CINEREA

Butternut, related to Walnut, is a remedy that often produces puzzled expressions when mentioned in a teaching situation. To be an effective homoeopath it is essential to be aware of all the available possibilities. If you use one of these small remedies successfully even once it will have served you and your patient well. Very small remedies are easily lost in a big repertorisation, so it is important to have a good knowledge of their materia medica.

Characteristic Skin Symptoms

Eruptions on the scalp, eyelids, wrists, backs of hands and legs.
Eruptions in patches.
Pustules on the extremities.
Moist eruptions, scabs.

The Itch

Scratching ameliorates.
Worse from becoming warm in bed.
Wandering itch.

Characteristic Mental Symptoms

Not likely to be many, but may exhibit mental fatigue, confusion, poor memory.
Irritable children.

Most Useful General Symptoms

Exertion ameliorates.
Liver problems with diarrhoea and occipital headaches.

KALI SULPHURICUM

This remedy is included here to represent all the Kali salts, any of which can have eczema in their picture. Kali Sulphuricum is the one most likely to be helpful, possibly because of the sulphur element in the compound. All the Kalis, where there are mental symptoms, have a similar attitude to life – they are proper, unadventurous people, often rigid in their views. Kali Sulphuricum, because of its modalities and generalities, is most easily confused with Pulsatilla and Sulphur.

Characteristic Eczema Symptoms

Scaly, profuse desquamation, especially yellow scales.
Crusty eruption.
Moist yellow crusts.
Cracks.
Moist eruption, especially yellow discharge.
Suppurating eczema.

The Itch

Worse from warmth, especially warmth of bed.
Itching with burning.
Burning after scratching.

Characteristic Mental Symptoms

Proper, rigid, inflexible attitude.
Hurried and irritable.
Anxiety ameliorated in the open air.
Fear of death, falling, people.
Worse from consolation.

Most Useful General Symptoms

Worse from warmth.
Better in the open air.
Worse from warmth but draughts aggravate (Sulphur).
Tendency to suppuration.
Aversion to eggs, fats, fish, meat and warm things.
Desires sweets.
Better from motion, especially in the open air.

112

LACHESIS

The best known of the snake remedies, Lachesis, needs little introduction. However, it has been used in situations, especially in infants, where the usually prominent mental symptoms were not apparent. In the realm of dermatology it is known more for ulcers than eczema, but like all the great polychrests it can be curative in a wide variety of physical manifestations of disease. Whenever Lachesis is indicated the other snake remedies should be borne in mind. Remedies such as Elaps, Naja, Vipera and so on may not feature as highly as Lachesis in a repertorisation and can easily be overlooked.

Characteristic Eczema Symptoms

The appearance is often suggestive: bluish or blackish discoloration; circumscribed pigmentation where eruption was; eruptions on hairy parts.
Blotches, cracks, crusts, vesicles, pustules (black), suppuration.
Discharge, usually bloody, after scratching.
Fetid eruptions.
Dry, inactive skin.
Suppressed eruptions.
Eczema alternating with asthma.
Eczema in the spring.
Swelling of the affected area.
Skin thickens after scratching.

The Itch

Worse at night.
Must scratch until raw.
Scratching aggravates.
Itching without eruption.
Worse for becoming heated.

Characteristic Mental Symptoms.

Loquacious, extrovert, passionate, exuberant.
Suspicious, jealous, envious.
Mentally active, good memory, theorising.
Religious, superstitious.
Fanaticism.
Fear of snakes.

113

Most Useful General Symptoms

Hot, worse for becoming heated and in warm rooms.
Worse on waking and from long sleep.
Left-sided.
Better for discharges.
Worse in humid weather, spring and summer.
Purplish discoloration.
Worse before menses and during menopause.

LYCOPODIUM

It is well known that Lycopodium and Sulphur are closely related. Their skin symptoms are virtually indistinguishable. It is rare to prescribe Lycopodium where there is not either an emotional aetiology or an emotional component to the case. Where infants exhibit Lycopodium symptoms it is often a state which they have inherited from their mother.

Characteristic Eczema Symptoms

Eruptions with concomitant urinary, gastric or hepatic troubles.
Crusty eruptions.
Moist fetid crusts, or dry but bleeding or discharging after scratching.
Eruptions on perspiring and hairy parts.
Cracks.

The Itch

Worse in the evening.
Worse on perspiring parts.
Must scratch until it is raw.
Worse from warmth.

Characteristic Mental Symptoms

Haughty, arrogant, dictatorial. These types of behaviour are usually only in situations where they feel safe and are a compensation for the following underlying emotions:
Lack of confidence, cowardice.
Intellectual type.
Intolerant of contradiction.
Fear of responsibility and anything new.

Tendency to anticipatory anxiety.
Helplessness.
Anxiety about health.

Most Useful General Symptoms

Worse 4–8 p.m.
Right-sided or right then left.
Worse for pressure of clothes.
Worse for warmth but draught aggravates.
Desires sweets, olives, warm food and drink.
Averse to beans and peas, oysters.
Onions, oysters, cabbage aggravate.
Worse on waking.
Worse for fasting.

MANGANUM

This is a remedy that can masquerade as several others, for example
Mercurius, Natrum Muriaticum and Sulphur, and will therefore often
be overlooked. It ranks somewhere between the small remedies and
the polychrests and has a distinctive picture that is important to be
aware of.

Characteristic Skin Symptoms

Painful cracks, especially in flexures.
Worse in winter.
Blotches and patches.
General sensitiveness of skin.
Poor healing, suppuration.
Eruptions in bends of joints.
Worse from sea bathing.

The Itch

Worse on perspiring parts and from perspiration.
Warmth can aggravate or ameliorate.
Scratching can aggravate or ameliorate.
Wandering itch.
Must scratch until raw.

Characteristic Mental Symptoms

Reserved, gloomy demeanour. Sulky.
Hatred, revengeful.
Grief.
Music aggravates.
Aversion to company and conversation.
Disposed to frown.

Most Useful General Symptoms

Lying down ameliorates.
Affinity for the ears, larynx and periosteum.
Allergic to feathers.
Worse for damp.
Worse at night.

MEDORRHINUM

Medorrhinum is not listed in the 'Eczema' rubric in the *Complete Repertory*, but like all the nosodes can play a part in its treatment. It is probably not needed as often as Psorinum and Tuberculinum, but should be remembered in sycotic cases where there is either moist eczema or itching with no eruption, even if it does not feature much in the repertorisation. It has the interesting feature of itching that is worse at night, for which it may not be thought of because of its well known general night-time amelioration.

Characteristic Eczema Symptoms

Allergic eczema.
Fetid, crusty eruption.
Reddish discoloration remains after eruption disappears.
Bleeding eczema.
Eruptions worse before and during menses.

The Itch

Worse in the evening and at night.
Rubbing gently ameliorates.
Unchanged by scratching.
Itch without eruption.
Thinking of it aggravates.
Undressing aggravates.

Characteristic Mental Symptoms

Extremes of mood and behaviour.
Hurry, time passes too slowly.
Anticipatory.
Feels in a dream, detached from reality.
Bites nails.
Clairvoyance.
Selfish, egotistical.
Weeps telling symptoms.
Fear of the dark, being alone at night, someone behind him, misfortune, insanity.
Weakness of memory.

Most Useful General Symptoms

Daytime aggravation.
Better lying on abdomen.
Better being fanned and from fresh air.
Better or worse from damp.
Better by the seaside.
Worse before and during storms.
Desires sweets, salt, fat, alcohol, fish, green fruit, ice, oranges.
Averse to aubergine, slimy food, sweets.

MERCURIUS SOLUBILIS

This has been one of the author's most frequently prescribed and useful remedies in the treatment of eczema, which begs the question 'Why?'. Could there be a link with dental amalgam? Mercurius appears in 458 rubrics in the 'Skin' section of the *Complete Repertory*. Whatever the reasons, its effect can be profound in some of the most severe cases, particularly when there is very intense itching that is worse at night and from warmth.

Characteristic Eczema Symptoms

Moist and bleeding eruptions.
Bleeding after scratching.
Foetid, offensive odour from the eruption, even if the discharge is scanty.
Thick crusts, vesicular or pustular eruption.
Deep, bloody cracks.
Worse in winter.

Worse on hairy parts.
Discharge destroys hair.
Ulceration and suppuration.

The Itch

Can be very intense and distressing.
Worse in evening and at night.
Warmth aggravates.
Wool aggravates.
Perspiration aggravates.
Undressing aggravates.
Scratching may ameliorate or aggravate.
Must scratch until raw.
Itch without eruption.

Characteristic Mental Symptoms

Keynotes of instability and oversensitivity.
Closed, unconfident people.
Delusion that everyone is an enemy. Easily offended.
Stammering.
Violent impulses.
Internal hurried feeling with slowness of execution.
Anarchist, disobedience, defiance.

Most Useful General Symptoms

Worse at night.
Worse from perspiration and easy perspiration.
Worse on becoming heated, or heat and cold aggravates.
Sensitive to weather changes and draughts.
Offensiveness.
Glandular affections, salivation.
Worse lying on right side.
Trembling and restlessness.
Desire for bread and butter, lemons.
Aversion to sweets, coffee, salt, fat.

MEZEREUM

A remedy that shares symptoms in common with Sulphur, not least in that its main affinity is the skin. It is one of the most essential eczema remedies, with a picture that is relatively easy to recognise.

Characteristic Eczema Symptoms

Crusts and scabs with purulent matter underneath.
Also pustules and vesicles and desquamation.
Eruptions alternating with asthma.
Washing aggravates.
Worse in winter.
Eczema after vaccination.
Often eruptions on the face, around eyes and mouth.
Bleeding after scratching.

The Itch

Intense itch.
Worse in the evening and at night.
Worse from warmth, better cool (although generally very chilly).
Itch without eruption.
Burning.
Scratching usually aggravates but may scratch until raw for relief.
Itch changes place on scratching, wanders.
Undressing aggravates.

Characteristic Mental Symptoms

Anxiety felt in the stomach.
Anticipatory.
Indifference.
Desire for company.

Most Useful General Symptoms

Worse at night.
Worse from suppressions.
Lack of vital heat (although skin worse for warmth).
Affinity for nerves and bones.
Effects of vaccination.
Herpetic tendency.
Desires fat, ham, bacon.

NATRUM MURIATICUM

This polychrest is familiar to all homoeopaths, especially for its use in the effects of grief. Needless to say, there is sure to be an emotional component to the case if this remedy is indicated. All the Natrum salts can have eczema in their pictures, and sometimes differentiating between them is not easy. The skin symptoms are similar in each of them.

Characteristic Eczema Symptoms

Mostly affects the margins of the hair, eyelids, around mouth, hands and flexures.
Raw, red inflamed eczema.
Crusty eruption with corrosive discharge.
Eruptions on hairy and perspiring parts.
Worse at the seaside and from excessive salt.
Worse from the sun and exertion.
Tendency to urticaria and vesicular eruptions.
Chapping and cracking of the skin.
Dryness, inability to perspire.
Greasy skin.
Worse before menses.

The Itch

Worse from exertion.
Worse from perspiration.
Worse from touch.
Worse undressing.
Worse from wool.

Characteristic Mental Symptoms

Ailments from grief and disappointment. Silent grief.
Desire to be alone yet fear of rejection. Self-reliant.
Dwells on past disagreeable occurrences. Resentful.
Avoids causing and being hurt. Defensive.
Sympathetic.
Guilt.
Consolation aggravates.
Closed, reserved and serious.

Most Useful General Symptoms

Worse from the heat of the sun.
Worse with the sun.
Worse or better by the seaside.
Worse 9–11 a.m.
Periodicity.
Worse from sympathy.
Better in the open air.
Desires salt, bitter, bread, fish, oysters, chocolate, coffee.
Aversion to salt, fat, coffee, fish, bread, chicken, slimy.

NITRIC ACID

This remedy can look like Natrum Muriaticum, especially in its emotional symptoms. The skin produces symptoms that may be very characteristic and instantly recognisable, or they may be more subtle and resemble those of related remedies like Graphites, Hepar Sulphuris, Mercurius, Petroleum, Sepia and Sulphur.

Characteristic Eczema Symptoms

Deep, bloody cracks.
Bleeding after scratching.
Painful eczema, especially burning and splinter-like pains.
Sensitive eruptions, e.g. to touch.
Eczema around the anus and genitals.
Eruptions on hairy parts.
Eruptions, especially crusts, in patches.
Discharging after scratching – corrosive or pus.
Fetid, offensive eruption.

The Itch

Cold air aggravates
Must scratch until it bleeds.
Itch changes place on scratching.
Undressing aggravates.
Warmth ameliorates.

Characteristic Mental Symptoms

Anxiety about health, fear of death.
Resentful, hatred, bitter, revengeful, litigious.

Dwells on past disagreeable occurrences. Tormenting thoughts.
Anger with cursing.
Discontented.
Quarrelsome.
Sensitive to all external impressions.
Selfish.

Most Useful General Symptoms

Worse from slight causes.
Worse for touch, jarring, noise.
Coldness.
Better for gentle motion.
Splinter-like pains.
Strong urine.
Affinity for angles and mucocutaneous margins.
Desires fat, salt, lime, fish.
Averse to cheese, meat.

OLEANDER

This small remedy is known mostly as a skin remedy although it also
has an affinity for the digestive tract.

Characteristic Skin Symptoms

Main affinity is the scalp, especially the back of the head.
Crusty discharging eruptions.
Cracks, desquamation and vesicles.
Very sensitive or painless eruptions.
Dryness, inability to perspire.
Numbness after scratching.
Skin chafes easily.

The Itch

Worse in cold air.
Worse at night.
Must scratch until it is raw.
Scratching aggravates or ameliorates.
Undressing aggravates.
Wandering itch.

Characteristic Mental Symptoms

Confusion, difficult concentration, as if in a dream.
Irritable, disposition to contradict.

Most Useful General Symptoms

Worse from oranges.
Sensation of emptiness.
General weakness and dullness.
Worse after suckling.
Ascending heights aggravates.
Acids aggravate.
Desires alcohol, potatoes.
Aversion to cheese.

PETROLEUM

Petroleum is very much a skin remedy, and is rarely used for anything else other than seasickness. It is one of the more easy skin remedies to identify and can help the most severe and distressing forms of eczema.

Characteristic Skin Symptoms

Deep, bloody cracks.
Eruptions worse in winter.
Terrible dryness.
Eruptions bleed after scratching.
Crusts, discharging after scratching.
Offensive suppurating eruptions.
Excoriation, burning.
Suppressed eczema.
Affects the occiput, folds, genitals, face and hands.
Skin heals with difficulty.
Rough, hard, thickened skin.

The Itch

Worse at night.
Worse in the open air.
Must scratch until raw.
Burning, smarting.
Warmth ameliorates.
Itching of orifices.

Characteristic Mental Symptoms

Irritable, fiery temperament (but not necessarily).
Quarrelsome, scolding. Ailments from anger.
Confusion – 'Loses way in well-known streets', sense of duality.
Irresolution, forgetful, discouraged.
Timidity, aversion to company.

Most Useful General Symptoms

Worse in winter.
Worse riding in a car or on a boat – general travel sickness.
Lack of vital heat, better in warm air.
Offensive perspiration.
Diarrhoea only in the daytime.
Worse after vexation.
Averse to fat and meat.
Desires beer and sweets.
Worse from cabbage, beans, flatulent food.

PHOSPHORUS

Phosphorus must be the most easy remedy in the materia medica to recognise, and also one of the most overprescribed. It is easy to be misled into thinking that every extrovert patient with a twinkle in their eye needs it. It is an important eczema remedy but the skin symptoms will mostly support your reasons for prescribing Phosphorus rather than suggesting it in their own right.

Characteristic Eczema Symptoms

Washing aggravates.
Blotches and patches.
Burning, stinging pains.
Desquamation, scaliness.
Vesicles and moist crusty eruptions.
Eruptions after scratching.
Tension of the skin.
Swelling of affected part.

The Itch

Worse at night and during sleep.
Must scratch until it is raw or until it bleeds.
Scratching usually ameliorates.
Undressing aggravates.
Wool aggravates.

Characteristic Mental Symptoms

Open, expressive people; extrovert, love company and relating.
Affectionate, tactile. Consolation ameliorates.
Fear of the dark, ghosts, being alone, disease, cancer, thunder.
Sympathetic, anxiety for others.
Feelings can be superficial – 'Out of sight, out of mind'.
Selfish even though sympathetic.
Becomes indifferent to loved ones when 'burnt out'.

Most Useful General Symptoms

Worse from slight causes.
Worse lying on the left side.
Worse from warm food.
Sensitive to weather and temperature changes.
Better for short afternoon sleep.
Better for rubbing, physical contact.
Desires spicy, salt, cold things, fish, ice cream, wine, chocolate.
Aversion to warm food and drink, tomatoes, fish, milk, sweets, vegetables, fruit.

PSORINUM

Psorinum has a particular affinity for the skin. Its rather extreme mental symptoms, as described in the old literature, do not need to be present for the remedy to be indicated. The most common mental symptom is its 'forsaken feeling', which may only express itself mildly. It should be remembered as an intercurrent remedy perhaps only needed during one stage of the treatment, especially where there is a history of suppression of the eruption. Occasionally it is the only remedy required to effect a dramatic improvement in atopic eczema. These are usually one-sided cases without Psorinum mental symptoms.

Characteristic Skin Symptoms

Eczema behind the ears and in the folds of skin generally.
Dirty-looking skin with poor healing.
Offensive discharges. Pus.
Crusts and vesicles.
Deep, bloody cracks, worse in winter.
Dryness, inability to perspire.
Eruptions alternating with respiratory symptoms.
Bleeding after scratching.
Cold air aggravates, and being overheated aggravates.
Eruptions in the spring and winter.
Washing aggravates.
Poor healing.

The Itch

Worse at night.
Worse for warmth of the bed.
Bleeding after scratching.
Itch without eruption.
Must scratch until it is raw or bleeds.
Undressing aggravates.
Warmth usually aggravates but sometimes ameliorates.
Wool aggravates.

Characteristic Mental Symptoms

Forsaken feeling.
Hopeless despair and pessimistic outlook on life,.
Fear of poverty.
Underfunction manifests in many ways: no ambition, willpower,
energy, love, success, faith etc.
Many anxieties. Forebodings.
Dull, difficulty thinking.
Despair from itching.

Most Useful General Symptoms

Very chilly.
Worse in winter.
Heat and cold aggravate.
History of suppressions.
Foul discharges.

Lack of reaction and recurrence of complaints.
After-effects of acute disease.
Feels well before an attack.
Worse from the approach of a storm.
Better for eating. Constant hunger.
Aversion to tomatoes, pork.

PULSATILLA

It is interesting that in Kent's *Repertory*, and even in modern repertories like the *Complete Repertory*, Pulsatilla does not appear in the Eczema rubric. It is the author's experience that it is not often successful on its own in eczema cases, and that if it seems indicated it is probably masquerading as another remedy. This is not a strict rule however, and as can be seen from the skin symptoms below it does have some characteristic eczema symptoms. When it is required it will probably be one of a sequence of remedies including deep-acting antipsorics like Calcarea Carbonica, Silicea or Sulphur, rather than being the single curative one.

Characteristic Skin Symptoms

Cracks, including deep bloody ones.
Chapping and dry burning.
Allergic eruptions.
Eruptions after scratching.
Eruptions on perspiring parts.
Eruptions on the back of the hands.

The Itch

Burning and prickling.
Must scratch until it is raw or bleeds.
Worse on perspiring parts.
Scratching aggravates or unchanged by scratching.
Wandering itch.
Wool aggravates.
Warmth aggravates.

Characteristic Mental Symptoms

Forsaken feeling.
Dependent people.
Mild, affectionate, easily moved to tears.
Consolation ameliorates.
Submissive, eager to please to gain favour and through fear of rejection.
Fastidious, sensitive to moral impressions.
Fear in a narrow place, being alone, darkness, insanity, at twilight, dogs, men.
Self-pity.
Envy and jealousy.

Most Useful General Symptoms

Worse from warmth.
Desire for open air, which ameliorates.
Worse at beginning of motion.
Worse in the evening.
Worse getting feet wet.
Worse at puberty, during pregnancy and before menses.
Better for a good cry.
Better for gentle motion.
Tendency to thick yellowish green discharges.
Worse lying on the left side.
Tendency to varicose veins.
Thirstlessness.
Desires cold food, eggs, ice cream, tea, spicy, bread and butter.
Averse to fats, butter, eggs, fruit, warm things, meat, pork, tobacco.
Worse from fat, pork, bread, butter, pastry, warm food, tobacco.

RHUS TOXICODENDRON

This is another remedy which, when well indicated, is fairly easy to recognise owing to its clear characteristic general and particular symptoms. It is one of the remedies that can be eliminated on the basis of the presence of one symptom – itching that is worse from warmth and better for cold – because of its very strong modality of being better from heat.

Characteristic Eczema Symptoms

Vesicular and crusty eruptions.
Eruptions alternating with internal affections.
Cold air aggravates.
Worse in the winter, spring and from change of weather.
Worse on perspiring parts.
Corrosive discharge.
Fissures, worse after washing.
Eruptions after scratching.
Swelling of affected part.
Eruptions around genitals and of hairy parts.
Hardness, thickening and inelasticity.
Tendency to urticaria and herpes.

The Itch

Better for warmth and worse in cold air.
Better for hot bathing.
Worse on hairy parts.
Worse from perspiration and on perspiring parts.
Scratching can aggravate or ameliorate.
Wool aggravates.

Characteristic Mental Symptoms

Restless, especially at night.
May come across as rather stiff, narrow-minded people.
Dwells on the past, especially at night.
Superstitious, fearful of ghosts, death, people being hurt.
Forsaken feeling.
'Causeless' weeping.
Wants to go home.
Anxiety about business.

Most Useful General Symptoms.

Worse from cold damp and exposure to cold.
Worse for uncovering.
Worse after midnight.
Worse at beginning of motion.
Better for continued motion, change of position, stretching.
Better from heat.
Desire for milk, oysters, sweets.

129

RHUS VENENATA

This remedy is similar to Rhus Toxicodendron but with a 'smaller' picture – for example, a skin case that has strong Rhus Toxicodendron skin symptoms but lacks the general symptoms such as the desire for milk or aggravation from damp. It may also have rheumatic symptoms.

Characteristic Eruption and Itch Symptoms

Itching better from hot bathing.
Eruptions worse in the cold air.
Vesicular eruptions, especially in groups.
Intense itch, worse at night.
Scratching aggravates.
Wandering itch.

SARSAPARILLA

Sarsaparilla has deep bleeding cracks like Petroleum. The cracks can be anywhere, including the hands, but a characteristic of this remedy is cracks on the feet. It has many sorts of eruptions apart from eczema in its picture – see the 'Skin' section of the repertory – psoriasis, boils, ulcers, pimples, warts, rashes, blotches, urticaria etc. One of the main remedies for cystitis where the pain is worst as the last few drops of urine are passed. It is mainly a sycotic remedy, as is evident from its bladder and wart symptoms.

Characteristic Skin Symptoms

Deep cracks.
Worse in the spring and summer, as markedly as Petroleum's winter aggravation.
Worse before and during menses.
Eruptions that date from vaccination.
Worse from washing.
Eruptions in patches and blotches.
Shrivelled-looking skin.

The Itch

It can have all four of the reactions to scratching: worse, better, changes place or unchanged.
Itch worse from warmth; worse at night and in the morning.

Characteristic Mental Symptoms

Changeable moods.
Forsaken feeling.
Offended easily.
Cheerful.
Dullness; mental exhaustion.

Most Useful General Symptoms

Worse at close of urination.
Worse in spring.
Worse at night.
Worse for cold damp.
Suppressed gonorrhoea.
Marasmus.
Gouty tendency.

SEPIA

Sepia is one of the most frequently indicated remedies for eczema. As one would expect, it is usually required where there are concomitant hormonal problems. Sepia eczema is most frequently, although not exclusively, seen in women and is the main remedy for eczema during pregnancy and lactation. It should not, however, be forgotten for eczema in childhood.

Characteristic Eczema Symptoms

Mostly on the face, occiput and bends of the joints.
Cracks that are worse for washing and in winter.
Eruptions on perspiring parts.
Worse in winter.
Dry or moist eczema. Dry, with yellow discharge after scratching.
May have pustules, vesicles or crusts.
Worse before menses, during pregnancy and lactation.
Hard thickening of the skin.
Swelling of the affected part.

The Itch

Worse in the open air.
Burning after scratching.

Must scratch until raw.
Scratching may aggravate or ameliorate.
Itch better from warmth but may be worse from warmth of bed.
Undressing aggravates.

Characteristic Mental Symptoms

Indifference to loved ones. Unaffectionate.
Worn out from cares.
Aversion to company.
Weeps telling symptoms.
Occupation ameliorates.
Consolation aggravates.
Defensive and critical.
Irritable before menses.
Fear of poverty.

Most Useful General Symptoms

Occupation ameliorates.
Exertion, dancing ameliorates.
Aversion to coition.
Very chilly, better for warmth but averse to stuffiness.
General physical stasis, dragging, bearing down, heavy sensations.
Left-sided.
Worse before menses and during pregnancy.
Worse around 5–6 p.m.
Desires chocolate, pickles, vinegar, spices, alcohol, sweets.
Averse to fat, meat, smell of food, salt.

SKOOKUM CHUCK

This remedy is included because it is unknown to many homoeopaths and has proved useful to the author. It is made from the water of Medical Lake in the USA so, like Carlsbad, Sanicula, Wiesbaden and others, is a natural 'combination remedy' containing many minerals and compounds. It is thought of as a specific for dry eczema after vaccination. The only other indication is hayfever-like sneezing with profuse coryza. It has no other guiding symptoms of use and is the sort of remedy only likely to be used when the more obvious ones have failed in cases of eczema after vaccination.

STAPHYSAGRIA

A Staphysagria eczema case will always have an emotional component to it, with the well known 'ailment from suppressed anger' being the most likely underlying cause of the skin problems. Where there is the possibility of more than one remedy – say, Ignatia, Natrum Muriaticum and Staphysagria – careful examination of the skin symptoms can yield a useful differentiation.

Characteristic Eczema Symptoms

Moist crusty eruptions.
Eruptions after scratching.
Offensive discharge.
Suppressed eruptions.
Eruptions in patches.
Scabs on the scalp.
Unhealthy skin, easily suppurating.

The Itch

Crawling as from insects. Tingling and prickling.
Worse in the cold air. Warmth ameliorates.
Itch changes place on scratching or is aggravated by scratching.
Wandering itch.
Undressing aggravates.

Characteristic Mental Symptoms

Ailments from suppressed emotions, especially anger.
Ailments from grief, wounded honour, embarrassment, indignation, rudeness of others, reproaches, mortification.
History of physical or emotional abuse.
Sensitive to discord and easily offended.
Mild and yielding temperament.
Conscientious about trifles.
Masturbation, sexually-minded.

Most Useful General Symptoms

Worse from sexual excess.
Generally worse from emotions.
Worse for touch.
Systemic effects of wounds, especially lacerated wounds.

Worse from tobacco.
Averse to milk, cheese.
Desires sweets, spicy, tobacco, soup, milk, rice.

SULPHUR

Sulphur is the king of polychrests and the best known 'skin remedy'. It is also the most overprescribed remedy, as it is easy to make Sulphur fit almost any situation in which there is an eruption. It can be partially similar to many cases, resulting in aggravation without amelioration.

It rarely has no effect at all on eczema. Probably the easiest way of convincing sceptics that medicines diluted beyond Avogadro's Constant have a real effect would be to give a group of eczematous sceptics Sulphur 200c for a few days! It is very much in the category of the 'unsuppressors' – it has a particularly powerful centrifugal action, in that it brings symptoms to the surface. It should be used with care where there is a history of suppression, or if the likelihood of similarity is low.

Characteristic Skin Symptoms

Itch worse from warmth.
Eruption worse from water.
Itch worse at night. (Can also be worse morning and evening.)
Eruption bleeding after scratching.
Cracking, worse from water and in winter.
Redness.
Itching with burning.
History of suppressed eruptions.
Eruptions alternating with respiratory complaints.
Eczema dating back to vaccination.

The Itch

One of the remedies for itch without eruption.
Alternates with burning. The burning is better while itching and the itching is relieved when the burning is worse.
Worse on perspiring parts.
Must scratch until raw.
Mostly worse for scratching but can be better for scratching.

Worse at night and during sleep.
Worse undressing.
Worse from wool.

Characteristic Mental Symptoms

Theorising, intellectual.
Selfish, egotism.
Critical.
Lazy, tendency to take short cuts.
May have: disgust, fastidiousness, anxiety for others; fear of heights, failure, narrow places, disease; hoarding, avarice.

Most Useful General Symptoms

Worse from warmth, desire for air but worse from draughts.
Uncovers feet.
Worse for bathing.
Worse from suppression, and a history of suppressions.
Hungry at 11 a.m.
Stoop-shouldered.
Offensiveness.
Desires chocolate, spices, fat, alcohol, sweets, apples, ice cream.
Averse to eggs, fish, sweets, vegetables.

A Note about Rubric Differentiation

Compare the following rubrics:

1) SKIN; ITCHING; bleeding; scratching, after
2) SKIN; ERUPTIONS; bleeding; scratching, after
3) SKIN; ITCHING; scratch; must; until it bleeds
4) SKIN; ITCHING; scratch; must; until it is raw

- The first two are interchangeable; they contain the same remedies.

- Rubrics (2) and (3) are *different*. Number (2) describes the nature of the eruption after scratching and number (3) is a modality of the itching. Number (3) is a smaller rubric and describes a symptom characteristic of Alumina, Arsenicum and Psorinum.

- Numbers (3) and (4) are different. The two rubrics describe a different group of remedies. Choosing between them should be done with care and is not always easy.

THUJA OCCIDENTALIS

Thuja, one of the most mysterious and difficult remedies to grasp, reveals little more of itself in its skin symptoms than it does by any other means. Of all the remedies it is probably the one most often prescribed 'on a hunch' or on the basis of a few keynotes. Some believe Thuja to be a remedy that almost everyone needs at some point in view of the smallpox vaccine miasm and Thuja's reputation for undoing its damage. It may be required for a certain stage in the treatment of eczema or may be the curative remedy.

Characteristic Eczema Symptoms

Eruptions on covered parts and perspiring parts.
Crusty, dry or discharging eruptions.
Vesicles, pimples and urticaria.
Eruptions in patches.

The Itch

Worse in the evening and at night.
Itching without eruption.
Itching on perspiring parts.
Scratching ameliorates.

Characteristic Mental Symptoms

Reserved, private, even secretive people.
Present a confusing, nebulous case history.
Fixed ideas, maybe in the form of fanaticism of some sort.
Questioning, doubtful, sceptical minds.
Motivated by presenting a perfect image to the world.
Perfectionism, fastidious.
Sensitive to music.
Hurried.

Most Useful General Symptoms

Worse from cold damp.
Ailments from vaccination.
Left-sided.
Ailments from suppressed and apparently cured STD.
Worse at 3 a.m. and 3 p.m.
Tendency to warts, growths and excrescences.

Oily skin.
Sweet perspiration.
Sweat on uncovered parts.
Desires salt, tobacco, onions.
Averse to onions, meat, tobacco, potatoes.
Worse from tea, fat, onions, potatoes.

TUBERCULINUM

Tuberculinum is often indicated in infantile eczema. Apart from the well known mental and general symptoms there are some useful guiding skin symptoms. Tuberculinum Koch is usually the favoured version of the remedy in skin conditions, but it may sometimes be necessary to compare the action of Tuberculinum Bovinum if Koch is not working as well as you might expect.

Characteristic Eczema Symptoms

Circinate eruptions.
Eczema from allergy to dairy produce.
Eczema with asthma or bronchitic tendency.
Rough, dry skin.
Eczema may be dry or discharging.
General erythema, red rash.

The Itch

Worse in the cold air.
Warmth ameliorates.
Itch ameliorated by tickling or stroking.
Worse at night.
Undressing aggravates.
Changes place on scratching.
Wandering itch.
Wool aggravates.
Touch sets off the itch.

Characteristic Mental Symptoms

Need for change and variety in life.
Frustrated, unfulfilled, discontented, romantic longings.
Desire to travel.

Fear of dogs and cats.
Restless, hyperactive children.
Destructive behaviour.
Optimistic.

Most Useful General Symptoms

Desire for open air.
Worse from cold damp.
Better or worse by the seashore.
Worse before storms.
Grinding of teeth during sleep.
Perspiration during sleep.
Ravenous appetite.
Desires meat, fat, bacon, salt, sweets, smoked things, delicacies, milk, ice cream.
Aversion to meat, eggs, milk.

VINCA MINOR

This little remedy is especially for crusty eruptions on the scalp which ooze offensive moisture and cause matting of the hair. The skin is very sensitive and becomes red and excoriated from slight friction. Foul crusty eruptions and burning, itching pustules.

VIOLA TRICOLOR

Wild Pansy is also used in herbal medicine for the treatment of eczema and it is likely that its homoeopathic use has its origins in herbalism.

Characteristic Skin Symptoms

Has a reputation as a remedy for eczema of childhood.
Affinity for the face and head.
Eczema with urinary symptoms.
Thick crusts and scabs exuding pus.
Cracking of the skin.
Eruptions in patches.
Eruptions after scratching.
Miliary eruptions.
Unhealthy skin.

The Itch

Scratching ameliorates.
Burning.
Itch worse at night.
Often an intense, intolerable itch.

Most Useful General Symptoms

Urine offensive, like cat urine.
Worse in winter.
Worse around 11 a.m.

Appendix

Essences and the Doctrine of Signatures

For the most part, the information given in this book is pragmatic and leans more towards the scientific than the artistic side of what we do. One of the most fascinating ways to study remedies is according to the Doctrine of Signatures. That is by studying, in great detail, the character of the material from which the remedy is made and seeing how the proving symptoms are a reflection of those physical characteristics.

By combining such a study with an analysis of the themes and patterns that run through the proving symptoms, it is possible to formulate an 'essence' for the remedy. This can be done for every remedy in the materia medica. The value of doing so is that it can go some way towards helping us to understand why a remedy produces particular symptoms in its picture. The remedy picture thus becomes more alive and cohesive – it makes more sense and is raised above the level of a mere list of symptoms. It is however a subjective exercise, rather like analysing literature, and because it involves individual perception and interpretation, is not always reliable or of practical use. This aspect of materia medica study has therefore deliberately been avoided in this book, but one example is included to illustrate the approach.

The cases mentioned below are not eczema patients and the aim here is to illustrate a way of studying remedies rather than to say anything particularly pertaining to eczema.

Kreosotum

Kreosotum or creosote (from the Greek meaning 'flesh preserver'). It is an oily liquid obtained by distillation of wood tar and pyroligneous acid, the preservative principle in smoke used for smoking meat and fish. It is also used to preserve wood. It is one of the several substances we use in homoeopathy which in its material form preserves dead organic matter and has the opposite effect on living tissue. It is a toxic substance causing gastroenteritis, vomiting, diarrhoea and eventually spasms, convulsions, coma and suffocation.

In the provings where the dynamic effects are brought out, the main characteristics of the remedy are a tendency to haemorrhages and the destruction of tissue; foul, acrid, excoriating discharges and burning pains, with a particular affinity for the mucous membranes of the female generative organs; malignant disease, abscesses, corrosion and erosion of the mucous membranes. The destructive tendency is also exhibited in the teeth symptoms, where they decay as soon as they appear.

So what we have is two extremes – flesh preserver and flesh destroyer. It is used to preserve wood, fish and meat, and in both its dynamic and material effect on the living we see the opposite destructive effect.

In each case where I have used Kreosotum successfully, the patient was in a situation where they were having to draw deeply on their survival instincts. What came through as a result of studying these cases together with the repertory, materia medica and provings, was a theme of self-preservation. My patients were all women, and in two cases struggling single parents in very insecure positions with great burdens of responsibility. One had ulceration of the cervix with haemorrhage and the other had arthritis of the left thumb (a keynote of this remedy). It is a strong symptom. Kreosotum is listed in black type with two other remedies in plain type only in the rubric 'Pain in the left thumb'. Looking at some of the other mental symptoms of the remedy there is something of a theme that supports this idea of being overburdened and in a survival situation.

Some of the sensations from the provings are:

As if a load resting on the pelvis
As if sternum crushed in
As if a heavy burden on the crest of the ileum
Sensations of internal and external constriction
Sensation of a tight band
As if small of back would break

The other fear the remedy has which, like the fear of coition, is a single symptom is 'Fear of fasting', and also in the picture is 'Worse from fasting'. Related to this is also the symptom 'Arrested development from nutritional disturbances'. The only other fear is 'Fear of impending disease'.

141

The dreams in the provings are the following:

Being poisoned
Emaciating
Something happening to her children
Being in open snow and being anxious about her children

While all of the above can be made to fit the idea I am presenting, I think this last dream is the real gem among them.

So what I am suggesting is that the remedy will be required either:

In situations where the flesh is being destroyed with the classic acrid putrid discharges, bleeding and ulceration and so on, or

In situations where flesh is being preserved in the figurative sense.

Think of the expression 'to save one's skin', which means to save one's life. Perhaps also the expression 'by the skin of one's teeth'. Situations of self-preservation. In such a case it seems there may or may not be physical flesh-destroying symptoms, but we would probably be reliant on some other Kreosotum keynotes in order to see the remedy – perhaps the desire for smoked things that the remedy shares with Calcarea Phosphorica and Causticum. Either way, from my experience so far, there is likely to be this theme of self-preservation in the person's life at the time that the remedy is required.

The keynote 'Fear of coition' can be interpreted as a fear of letting go of one's self, perhaps another symptom of too strong a need for self-preservation.

The teeth symptoms, too, are interesting. The keynote of teeth that begin to decay as soon as they appear – that stage of life represents the beginning of the emergence of the self-preservation instinct. There is a connection here to the other single symptom already mentioned – the fear of fasting, which can also be seen to be suggesting the same instinct.

It is also a remedy for teething infants with a similar picture to Chamomilla. Kreosotum has less of the anger, is less besides himself than Chamomilla. They both have the desire to be carried, but Kreosotum likes being caressed whereas Chamomilla has an aversion to being touched. Chamomilla likes to be rocked. They are both capricious. Above all, it is the early decay and blackness of teeth that is characteristic of Kreosotum. Even the menses can be excoriating and offensive.

Other Chief Symptoms

It affects the mucous membranes of the digestive tract to the same extent as the genitalia.

Erosion of the stomach with haematemesis.

Vomiting of undigested food that has been in the stomach for hours.

Hot eructations.

Bloody diarrhoea.

Cough with burning in the chest and haemoptasis.

Small wounds bleed freely.

Spongy bleeding gums.

Toothache during pregnancy.

Gangrene internally and externally.

Moist eczema that itches violently.

Very chilly and worse from cold food.

Worse in the open air and better from indoor air.

Premenstrual headaches.

Erosion of the cervix.

Kreosotum most resembles Arsenicum, Nitric Acid and Sulphur in its physical symptomatology.

GENERAL INDEX

REMEDY INDEX

RUBRIC INDEX

CHEST; ALTERNATING with; skin
symptoms, 8

EAR; ERUPTIONS;
eczema, 11
eczema; meatus, 12
behind the ears; moist, 77
EXTREMITIES; CRACKED skin; hands, 55
EXTREMITIES; ERUPTIONS;
ankle; eczema; varicosum, 10
joints; bends of, 64, 68
EXTREMITIES; ITCHING; lower limbs;
varices, 10
EXTREMITIES; NAILS; affections of;
exfoliation, 68
EXTREMITIES; VARICES; leg; itching, 10
EXTREMITIES; WALK; late learning to,
64
EYE; ERUPTIONS;
eyebrows, about, 12
lids, on; margins, 12
EYE; INFLAMMATION; lids; margins, 12

FACE; DISCOLORATION; red; circumscribed, 55

GENERALITIES; ALLERGY, 8
GENERALITIES; FANNED;
being; amel., 57
desire to be, 58
GENERALITIES; FOOD and drinks;
bananas; desires, 73
cheese; aversion to, 73
milk; desires, 64, 68
pungent things; desires, 62
salt or salty food; desires, 39
spices, condiments, piquant, highly
seasoned food; desires, 38, 54
sweets; desires, 64
GENERALITIES; HEAT;
sensation of, 26, 57
vital, lack of, 26, 63
GENERALITIES; HEATED, becoming, 57,
59

GENERALITIES; SEASONS; summer;
agg., 70
GENERALITIES; TOBACCO; desires;
smoking, 48
GENERALITIES; VACCINATION; after, 67
GENERALITIES; VEINS; varicose,
distended, engorged, plethoric;
itching, 10

HEAD; DANDRUFF, 11
HEAD; ERUPTIONS;
crusts, scabs, 7
itching, 59
milk crust, 11
HEAD; PERSPIRATION; scalp; sleep;
during, 54
HEAD; SEBORRHOEA, 11

MIND; ABRUPT, rough, 63
MIND; AILMENTS from;
admonition, 102
anger, vexation, 28
grief, sorrow, care, 28
love; disappointed, unhappy, 47
MIND; ALTERNATING mental and
physical symptoms, 26
MIND; ANSWERS;
hastily, 31
incorrectly, 31
irrelevantly, 31
monosyllabic, 31
slowly, 31
MIND; ANXIETY; trifles about, 62
MIND; BITING, 73
MIND; CHEERFULNESS, 48
MIND; CONSCIENTIOUS about trifles, 62
MIND; DELUSIONS; war, being at, 70
MIND; DISCONTENTED, displeased,
dissatisfied, 48, 73
MIND; DISCOURAGED, 48
MIND; ENVY, 48
MIND; FASTIDIOUS, 38, 54, 62
MIND; FEAR; noise, from, 64
MIND; FORSAKEN feeling, 39

150

SKIN; HARD (*continued*)
 thickening, with, 9
SKIN; INFLAMMATION, 70
SKIN; ITCHING;
 air; cold; agg., 54, 67
 bleeding; scratching, after, 67, 135
 eruption; without, 55, 59
 evening, 51
 hairy parts, 12
 morning; bed, in, 68
 night, 39, 44, 51, 52, 53, 54, 55, 57,
  63, 64, 77
 scratch; must; until it bleeds, 51,
  101, 135
 scratch; must; until it is raw, 51, 135
 scratching; amel., 52, 55
 scratching; changing place, on, 43,
  69

SKIN; ITCHING; (*continued*)
 undressing; agg., 52, 67
 wandering, 47, 69
 warm, becoming, 43, 51, 53, 54, 55,
  59, 67
 warmth; amel., 67
 wool; agg., 48, 52
SKIN; PAIN; scratching, after, 77
SKIN; SENSITIVENESS; sun, to, 8
SKIN; ULCERS; discharges; green,
  56
SLEEP; SLEEPLESSNESS; itching, from,
  67
SPEECH & VOICE; SPEECH;
 slow, 31
 stammering, 31

TEETH; DENTITION; difficult, 32